THE
SUGAR
DETOX
DIET
for 50+

A COMPLETE GUIDE TO
Quitting Sugar, Boosting Energy,
and Feeling Great

DR. DANA ELIA
DCN, MS, RDN

Published in the US by:
ULYSSES PRESS
PO Box 3440
Berkeley, CA 94703
www.ulyssespress.com

ISBN: 978-1-64604-149-7
Library of Congress Control Number: 2020946993

Printed in the United States by Kingery Printing Company
10 9 8 7 6 5 4 3 2

Acquisitions editor: Casie Vogel
Managing editor: Claire Chun
Project editor: Renee Rutledge
Proofreader: Anne Healey
Front cover design: Ashley Prine
Cover art: © Okrasiuk/shutterstock.com
Interior design: what!design @ whatweb.com
Interior art: page 12 sucrose © grebeshkovmaxim/shutterstock.com;
    page 17 person © Christos Georghiou/shutterstock.com; page 67
    scale © igorrita/shutterstock.com; page 85 bottles © Vector FX/
    shutterstock.com

This book has been written and published strictly for informational purposes, and in no way should it be used as a substitute for consultation with your medical doctor or health-care professional. All facts in this book came from medical files, clinical journals, scientific publications, personal interviews, published trade books, self-published materials by experts, magazine articles, and the personal-practice experiences of the authorities quoted or sources cited. You should not consider educational material herein to be the practice of medicine or to replace consultation with a physician or other medical practitioner. The author and publisher are providing you with information in this work so that you can have the knowledge and can choose, at your own risk, to act on that knowledge. The author and publisher also urge all readers to be aware of their health status and to consult health professionals before beginning any health program, including changes in dietary habits.

For all those who seek to regain the power over their body and what goes into it. Let us break free from the unhealthy foods that drive and define our choices.

CONTENTS

CHAPTER 8

RECIPES 148

PREFACE

As a clinical functional nutrition doctor and registered dietitian nutritionist, my goal for this book is to explain to those of you in the fifty and over crowd how to safely and effectively eliminate excess sugar from your diet to boost energy, help with weight loss, and prevent harmful health conditions such as heart disease, diabetes, and cognitive dysfunction. Unlike many other books on this topic, our journey together will focus on stepping down from a life driven by sugar, rather than an abrupt breakup. Inside, you'll also find recipes for breakfast, lunch, dinner, and snack options. Taming your sweet tooth has never been easier!

INTRODUCTION

Welcome—I'm so glad that you've chosen to take the initial step toward improving your health, and I look forward to providing you with some tools and resources to help you along your wellness journey. Together we're going to map out just whom this book is geared for and why it's important to take an honest look at your diet and relationship with sugar. I've been in these trenches myself, having struggled with sugar cravings, weight issues, and trying to navigate my way through determining what my body truly needs most in order to thrive and function optimally.

You may be curious about what makes me an expert on sugar, detoxing, or dieting, as it seems diet experts are a dime a dozen these days. If I told you I had been a dieter for decades, would that make me an expert? I've also gone from weighing well over 300 pounds, barely squeezing myself into a size 26, to maintaining a healthy weight in the 140s. Does successfully losing weight automatically make me an expert on the topic? It may seem like many of the pop culture experts are those who've tried a diet, were successful, and now suddenly have a platform to claim expertise in diet and nutrition. However, dieting success does not equate to expertise; therefore, I strongly encourage you to seek out nutrition and all health-related advice from qualified, licensed clinicians.

For most of my young adult life, weight management was an issue. I was born a big baby at 8 pounds 12 ounces. As a functional medicine provider, I can now recognize the factors that influenced my own health struggles and sparked decades of battling my weight. In fact, when teaching students or speaking to other clinicians, I often use my own timeline and matrix as the perfect example for a functional medicine case study. We are all dealt a hand of cards with which to play and, unfortunately, my hand was less than perfect. But it led me down a path that I am forever grateful for, as the struggle is often the most important part of each individual's journey. Mine has taught me many invaluable lessons.

The brief CliffsNotes version of my history includes exposure to various toxins in utero, being born via C-section, not being breastfed, experiencing food sensitivities that emerged at a young age (some still persist today), getting irritable bowel syndrome (IBS), and getting chronic strep infections that ultimately led to a diagnosis of juvenile rheumatoid arthritis. Thus began an onslaught of drugs and health issues through my elementary school, high school, and even college years. For years I was given various rounds of corticosteroids, high doses of aspirin, nonsteroidal anti-inflammatory drugs (NSAIDs), and eventually, Plaquenil and weekly methotrexate injections. By the time I was ready to begin my undergraduate program in dietetics, I was morbidly obese, and my rheumatologist had added hypothyroidism, fibromyalgia, and systemic lupus erythematosus to my diagnosis list, along with suggestions for more heavy-duty meds. Throughout my preteen, teenage, and even college years,

I experimented with every single diet imaginable and was even put on prescription diet pills. My decision to study nutrition and dietetics instead of going premed as I had always intended stemmed from being at my wit's end in the fight to heal my own body. I decided there had to be a better way than what conventional diets and allopathic, or traditional, conventional medicine had offered me.

That journey has taken me on the path of personal exploration and truly learning to be in tune with my body's signals. Along the way, I've not only successfully maintained a healthy weight and managed my autoimmune issues solely through nutrition and lifestyle, but also earned three degrees in health and nutrition. So back to the question of expertise in the field of nutrition: education combined with personal experience does in fact qualify me as a subject-matter expert. Diet and nutrition have been my life's passion as they have been the key to my personal health and wellness, as well as that of my patients.

When I did my undergraduate training in dietetics in the early 1990s, the approach to nutrition and health was very much in line with traditional conventional medicine dogma. That approach never quite sat well with me, not only because it didn't work for my own struggles with weight and autoimmune disease, but also because I had seen it fail friends and family time and time again. I was drawn early on in my studies to what we now call integrative and functional medicine. Over the past few years, I've been pleased to see more awareness and acceptance of more integrative and functional approaches to health, wellness, and chronic disease management.

After working in the fields of nutrition and dietetics for over twenty-five years, I feel as if we are finally at a crossroads where traditional allopathic providers and integrative and functional providers meet. Collectively, we are working with more knowledge and a better understanding of just how influential diet and nutrition are in chronic disease. For example, evidence-based research illustrates the complex issue of obesity. It is not merely a seesaw balancing calories in versus calories out; that's the old energy balance mentality. We will explore some of the factors contributing to the obesity epidemic in our discussions herein.

Our society is at a critical breaking point. The current generation will likely be sicker, with shorter life expectancies than their parents' generation. It's a frightening thought to imagine that our children will live shorter, unhealthier lives than we will. Obesity rates are spiraling out of control, along with other chronic health issues. For example, the rates of inflammatory bowel disease (IBD) have skyrocketed. The Western diet (or Standard American Diet—SAD), with its promise of inexpensive, quick fixes that taste good, is fueling this crisis. SAD's composition of highly refined carbohydrates, excessive sugar, chemical-laden and genetically modified foods, trans fats, and refined omega-6 vegetable oils makes it a highly combustible combination, existing merely to promote inflammation and illness.

As my membership card to the fifty and over club looms right around the corner, my goal is to help you see that food can be a powerful tool in making the fifties and beyond your best years yet! And the real kicker here is that these years do not need to be sugar-coated!

CHAPTER 1

WHAT'S THE 411 ON NUTRITION BASICS?

Let's get this journey underway. I'm going to challenge you by asking you to cast aside everything you think you know about nutrition and diet. What we do know beyond a shadow of a doubt is just how profound an impact a poor-quality diet has on our health. Such a diet consists of a higher intake of processed foods, resulting in an overall higher intake of calories but a loss of vital nutrients. Poor-quality diets are typically deficient in fiber, vitamins, minerals, essential fatty acids, and other healthy components such as polyphenols and other phytonutrients. Polyphenols and phytonutrients are obtained through plant-based foods. In my opinion, they are nature's miracle workers, as they are jam-packed with antioxidants and a multitude of health benefits. For our focus on sugar detox, phytonutrients help to stimulate enzymes that assist the body to get rid of toxins while also giving a boost to the immune system, promoting healthy metabolism of hormones (like estrogen), enhancing cardiovascular health, and hastening the death of cancer cells.

Now, I want you to take a moment to jot down some examples of your current typical food choices, your reasons for having purchased this book, what changes you are willing to make, and what your ultimate goals are. This will become helpful to you later on in the book as we explore your motivation and readiness to make changes, as well as create a vision with specific steps to reach your goals.

NUTRITION 101

Before we jump into the practical side of a "diet" or lifestyle changes, it's important to invest some time to review some fundamentals of food composition, chemistry, and even a bit of biochemistry. Depending on your interest in nutrition, this may seem more like a review, but as new research becomes steadily available, we can all benefit from a refresher from time to time. Plus, if you're like me and grew up as a Generation Xer or a baby boomer, most of what we were taught about diet, nutrition, and metabolism is grossly outdated and even negligently incorrect.

Remember the four food groups, or even worse, the dreadful Food Guide Pyramid? During the heyday of the Food Guide Pyramid, I often felt that the more people followed the recommended servings listed, the more their bodies began to resemble the shape of a pyramid. Setting some foundational nutritional guidelines here that put such misguided principles in context will help the content appearing later in the book make more sense. I promise to make it as simple and painless as possible. You'll only have one quiz to take, and you're the only one who will see the results!

The bottom line is to start reciting the word "balance." As we dive further into our journey, balance will be a constant theme. As with most things in life, the healthiest of situations are those that are in balance.

While we're going to spend much of our time dissecting carbohydrates and sugars, it's imperative to set the stage by including some tried-and-true nutrition basics. Nutrients in the foods we eat can be divided into two main categories: macronutrients and micronutrients. Carbohydrates, proteins, and fats make up the macronutrients group. Fat-soluble vitamins, water-soluble vitamins, microminerals, and trace minerals round out the micronutrients group. Macronutrients are the ones that our bodies need in the largest amounts. They also supply the body with energy in the form of calories. Carbohydrates and fats are the main fuel suppliers of caloric energy to the body, and protein is the body's main source of construction material in the form of amino acids.

A WHIRLWIND TOUR OF THE MACRONUTRIENTS

CARBOHYDRATES

Carbohydrates are divided into three groups: monosaccharides, disaccharides, and polysaccharides.

Monosaccharides are simple sugars. Only a handful of the monosaccharides found in nature can actually be absorbed, and thus used, by our bodies.

- **Glucose:** blood sugar, also called dextrose; an essential energy source; is part of every disaccharide and is the most important monosaccharide

- **Fructose:** fruit sugar, also called levulose; sweetest of the sugars

- **Galactose:** found in dairy

Note to remember: No matter how complex a carbohydrate starts off, once in the body, all carbohydrates (except fibers) are broken down into these three simple sugars: glucose, fructose, and galactose. Since our brains require a regular supply of glucose, our bodies have an intricate process for maintaining a necessary amount of brain fuel.

A QUICK GLANCE AT CARBS

- Carbs provide 4 calories per gram.
- Carbs are considered to be the body's preferred fuel source.
- They can be stored in the body for later use as energy.
- The liver and muscles store carbohydrates in the form of glycogen (although our body's main form of stored fuel is fat). Glycogen is a polysaccharide, which turns out to be stored sugar, as it is many glucose molecules connected together. More on the classifications of carbohydrates in a bit.
- Carbs are not just sugars to be demonized. They exist in three main forms: sugar, starch, and fiber.
- Plants are a source of carbohydrates. They are found in fruits, grains, vegetables, beans, legumes, and even nuts and seeds.
- Some dairy products, such as milk, kefir, and yogurt, contain carbohydrates.
- Carbohydrates spare protein to preserve the body's lean muscle mass.

Disaccharides are pairs of monosaccharides, each containing a glucose molecule that is paired with another of the three monosaccharides. Disaccharides come mainly from plants; however, lactose and one of its components, galactose, come from milk and milk products.

- **Maltose/malt sugar:** made from two glucose units. Maltose tastes less sweet than sucrose. It is the least common disaccharide found in nature. Mainly present in germinating grain (malt), it can also be found in a small proportion in corn syrup.

- **Sucrose/table sugar:** made from one unit of glucose and one unit of fructose. Sucrose is produced naturally in plants. Table sugar is the refined form of sucrose that we are all too familiar with. Sucrose is typically consumed in overabundance by most Americans as it is an additive found in many commercially processed foodstuffs.

- **Invert sugar:** a mixture of glucose and fructose in a 1:1 ratio. It is another natural form of sugar. Invert sugar is a thick, syrupy, liquid sweetener often used commercially because it is sweeter (by volume) than sucrose as the bonds between glucose and fructose have been broken.

- **Lactose/milk sugar:** made from one unit of galactose and one unit of glucose. Lactose is the naturally occurring sugar found in dairy products.

How do common sweeteners measure up to table sugar? The following chart is a list of naturally derived sweeteners ranked in order of their level of sweetness as compared to table sugar. They are listed by "sweetness value percentage," from less sweet to most sweet. We'll dig into the artificial ones later.

NATURALLY DERIVED SUGARS COMPARED TO TABLE SUGAR

NATURAL SUGAR	SWEETNESS VALUE PERCENTAGE
Lactose	16%
Maltose	32%
Galactose	32%
Mannitol	50%
Sorbitol	60%
Glucose	74%
Xylitol	100%
Sucrose	100%
Invert sugar	130%
Fructose, levulose	173%

Source: Data from the US Food & Drug Administration, "Food Ingredients & Packaging," updated July 30, 2020, https://www.fda.gov/food/food-ingredients-packaging, and Krause's Food & The Nutrition Care Process.

Polysaccharides are chains of monosaccharides and include glycogen, starches, and dietary fibers. Corn, arrowroot, rice, potatoes, and tapioca are just a few examples of starches in this category. Glycogen and starch are both stored forms of glucose. Glycogen is found in the human body, while starch is found in plants. Yet, both forms provide energy for human use. Dietary fibers also contain glucose as well as other monosaccharides; however, since our bodies do not possess the digestive enzymes needed to break apart their bonds, they yield little, if any, caloric energy. Functional fibers are nondigestible carbohydrates from plant sources that are extracted or manufactured. Both dietary fiber and functional fiber have numerous benefits, such as helping to keep the function of our GI tract in check and reducing the risk of certain diseases, including some cancers. Keep that fact tucked away; we'll chat more about fiber and how it can be our best friend later.

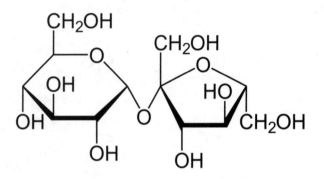

Chemical structure of sucrose.

Since we're going to be diving deep into both sugar and detoxing, we have to spend some time reviewing the process of carbohydrate digestion and absorption.

Carbohydrate Digestion and Absorption

Carbohydrate digestion begins with the mouth as enzymes in saliva (salivary amylase) start breaking down starches. The activity of amylase diminishes as carbohydrates reach the stomach due to stomach acid. In the stomach, carbohydrate digestion takes a backseat and proteins and fats begin to be broken down. As food continues its journey to the small intestine, carbohydrate digestion picks back up and the body breaks down starches into the disaccharide maltose. Maltose and the other disaccharides (lactose and sucrose) from foods we consume are broken down into monosaccharides, which our bodies absorb.

The majority of carbohydrate digestion and absorption occurs in the small intestine, thanks to the presence of the following enzymes: maltase, sucrase, lactase, and pancreatic amylase. Lactose intolerance is a common digestive issue that occurs when there is insufficient lactase to digest the disaccharide lactose, found in milk and milk products. According to the National Institutes of Health (NIH), approximately 65 percent of the world's population has a reduced ability to digest lactose after infancy.

Interestingly, lactose intolerance is actually determined by one's genes, and its prevalence is higher in some corners of the globe. The National Library of Medicine's Genetics Home Reference details the prevalence of lactose intolerance: in people of East Asian descent, 70 to 100 percent of adults can be affected. Additionally, lactose intolerance is often seen in people of West African, Arab, Jewish, Greek, and Italian descent. Lactose intolerance is lowest in populations where unfermented milk products, such as milk, ice cream, evaporated milk, and sweetened condensed milk, have historically been an important food source in the cultural diet. For example, less than 5 percent of those with Northern European ancestry are lactose intolerant. Those with lactose intolerance may be able to tolerate some fermented dairy products due to the action of the microbes aiding in the fermentation.

Lactose intolerance in infants (congenital lactase deficiency) is rare and is caused by mutations in the LCT gene. This gene provides instructions to the body for making the lactase enzyme. Lactose intolerance in adulthood is due to the gradually decreasing activity of the LCT gene. Adults whose LCT gene remains active (and thus can still produce lactase) are experiencing the benefit of a DNA-controlling sequence called a regulatory element, located within a nearby gene called MCM6. These "lucky" individuals have inherited changes in this element that result in a sustained lactase production in the small intestine and the ability to digest lactose throughout life, so they can continue to consume unfermented dairy without the side effects of lactose intolerance. I was the lucky one here: I can tolerate dairy well, but my brother cannot even look at it. But he trumps me in the gluten department, so the jury is still out on who got the raw deal in the dairy-gluten wars. That battle alone is fodder for many raging debates, as both can cause numerous GI and immune-related issues.

A few factors can impact our ability to digest carbohydrates. These include:

- The accessibility of the starch to enzymatic action; is the starch you eat being exposed to enough enzymes?
- The activity and availability of digestive enzymes in the upper GI tract; is there a sufficient amount of the enzymes being produced by the body to work on the starch you eat?
- The presence of fat or fiber in the GI tract, which can slow down digestion and give the enzymes more time to work on the starch you eat

Simple vs. Complex Carbs

The main key to success with carbs is being aware of the difference between simple and complex carbohydrates in the foods you choose to eat. Ideally, if you're eating in *balance,* digestion and absorption should slow the pace of glucose being released for delivery to the cells, in order to minimize the spike in blood glucose levels and the flood of insulin that results. Therefore, diets with plentiful whole foods such as minimally processed grains, nuts, seeds, legumes, non-starchy vegetables, and low-glycemic fruits will result in a slower rate of glucose absorption. After glucose is digested, it is actively absorbed across intestinal cells and then transferred in the portal bloodstream to the liver.

You may be familiar with trendy phrases like "quick" or "fast carbs" versus "slow carbs." Processed, refined, simple, naked carbs are the fast/quick ones, meaning there's not a whole lot of substance to them, making them quick and easy to break down and hit the bloodstream. Carbs, like life, should not be a race. Think the tortoise versus the hare. To be successful with long-term sugar detoxing, we'll be aiming for a slow, steady shift away from the fast carb lane. We'll talk more about what happens next to glucose in Chapter 2.

Why Fiber Can Be My New BFF

Fiber can be our friend for multiple reasons, and in the 50+ crowd, you definitely want to make fiber part of your inner circle! As we describe fiber's benefits below, reflect on how you may have been overlooking this key nutritional buddy. If you yearn to age gracefully, healthfully, and take steps to ensure longevity, fiber can no longer be excluded from your "in" crowd.

Fiber is commonly classified as either soluble, which dissolves in water, or insoluble, which doesn't dissolve. Fiber helps to regulate the passage of food through the digestive tract, which can aid in satiety. It influences the body's ability to control energy intake as it slows the absorption of glucose, so meals with higher fiber content will also help to prevent rapid shifts in blood glucose and insulin levels. Additionally, fiber can block the absorption of fats and cholesterol, which, combined with the slower absorption of sugars, can improve blood glucose and blood lipid levels. Fiber has also been shown to have an anti-inflammatory effect by decreasing blood levels of C-reactive protein (a marker for inflammation and heart disease risk) and proinflammatory cytokines that contribute to arterial plaques.

Fiber is the GI tract's cleaning crew, which also attracts water into the large intestine, helping to improve bowel function, an important part of the body's detoxification process (more to come on that topic later). Another important reason to maintain a proper intake of fiber is that it helps to feed your good gut bugs, and we know how much of an important role a healthy gut microbiome is to whole body health. By doing an analysis of an individual's microbiome, we can see how that individual's choice of carbohydrates and fiber have impacted the microbial diversity within their gut.

If you need some more reasons to be sure you are getting enough fiber, diets high in dietary fiber have been shown to decrease the rates of:

- heart disease
- stroke
- peripheral vascular disease
- hypertension
- diabetes
- hyperlipidemia
- obesity

In the battle of the bulge, both soluble and insoluble fiber can present a trifecta of benefits. They help keep us full and satisfied, but they contribute little, if any, caloric energy. By staying fuller longer, those who consume a high-fiber diet typically consume fewer simple carbohydrates and overall total calories, which can aid in weight loss or in maintaining a healthy body weight. Additionally, as soluble fiber is fermented in the large intestine, the satiety-inducing hormones glucagon-like peptide and peptide YY are created. Finally, dietary fiber can reduce the amount of energy available for your body to metabolize into caloric fuel, which is a bonus when trying to shed a few pounds.

Have you ever heard of certain foods being calorically neutral or calorically negative? Take celery, for instance. It takes the body more calories to digest and absorb the nutrients from celery than what celery actually yields.

CARBOHYDRATE DIGESTION IN THE BODY

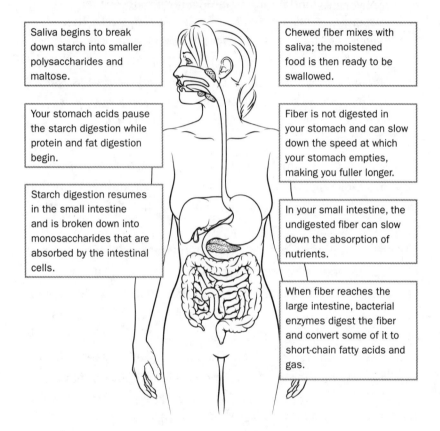

Saliva begins to break down starch into smaller polysaccharides and maltose.

Your stomach acids pause the starch digestion while protein and fat digestion begin.

Starch digestion resumes in the small intestine and is broken down into monosaccharides that are absorbed by the intestinal cells.

Chewed fiber mixes with saliva; the moistened food is then ready to be swallowed.

Fiber is not digested in your stomach and can slow down the speed at which your stomach empties, making you fuller longer.

In your small intestine, the undigested fiber can slow down the absorption of nutrients.

When fiber reaches the large intestine, bacterial enzymes digest the fiber and convert some of it to short-chain fatty acids and gas.

Remember, success with carbs is being mindful of the difference between simple and complex carbohydrates in your food choices. We discussed how they differ by chemistry and rate of digestion and absorption, and that makes all the difference when trying to "detox" from sugar.

PROTEINS

A QUICK GLANCE AT PROTEIN

- Protein provides 4 calories per gram.
- It is the workhorse of the cell.
- The body's construction material, protein is needed for structure, regulation, and function of the body's cells, tissues, and organs as well as metabolic, transport, and hormone systems.
- Proteins are a vital component of cell membranes. They can carry nutrients across the cell membrane and also serve as the messenger for signals from inside and outside of cells.

Proteins are more complex than carbohydrates or fats, AKA lipids, differing molecularly from the other two macronutrients in that they contain nitrogen. They also differ in their job description, which includes service duties such as structural protein, enzyme, hormone, transport protein, and immunoprotein. Protein can also be an energy source, yielding 4 calories per gram. While carbohydrates are made up of saccharides, proteins consist of amino acids linked together by peptide bonds. Proteins are made of some twenty different amino acids and classified as either essential, nonessential, or conditionally essential. The nine essential amino acids are the ones our body cannot make on its own and therefore must be obtained through diet. They are histidine, isoleucine, leucine, lysine, methionine, phenylalanine, threonine, tryptophan, and valine.

Nonessential means that our bodies produce these amino acids, regardless of whether we get them from the food we eat. The nonessential amino acids include alanine, arginine, asparagine, aspartic acid, cysteine, glutamic acid, glutamine, glycine, proline, serine, and tyrosine. Conditionally essential amino acids are usually not essential, except in times of illness and stress. These include arginine, cysteine, glutamine, glycine, tyrosine, proline, serine, and ornithine.

In situations where one's diet is low in carbohydrates or in starvation cases, a lack of glucose from food and depleted glycogen stores may result. Through the process of gluconeogenesis, which literally means "to create glucose," the body makes glucose from non-sugar sources such as lactate, pyruvate, and glucogenic amino acids. Of the twenty amino acids, lysine and threonine are the only two that the body cannot use to produce at least some amount of glucose. Instead, these two are often referred to as ketogenic amino acids since they create products that the body converts to ketones and uses for energy.

Throughout this book, I will stress the importance of the food quality. Digestibility is a major factor impacting protein quality. Some summary points to be aware of regarding protein quality and digestibility are:

- Meat preparation procedures intended to tenderize cuts of meat can make proteins more accessible to digestive enzymes. These enzymes break the proteins down into their simplest form—amino acids.

- Vegetable protein is less efficient than animal protein because it is enclosed by carbohydrate, which makes it less available to digestive enzymes.

- Some plants contain proteins called lectins that can interfere with protein digestion and must be inactivated by heat before consumption. They are mostly found in legumes, grains, and nightshade vegetables.

- Amino acids can be damaged by food processing.

- Food processing can reduce the digestive availability of amino acids, as well as other nutrients contained in the protein-containing food.

- Proper cooking and storing of protein foods is vital to maintain the quality and usefulness of the amino acids the source is intended to provide.

FATS

A QUICK GLANCE AT FATS

- Fats provide 9 calories per gram.
- An essential fuel source, fats support cell growth and protect organs.
- Fats aid in body temperature regulation and provide insulation.
- They also aid in the transportation and absorption of certain nutrients.
- Fats are necessary for the synthesis of hormones and neurotransmitters.

Fats and lipids make up about 34 percent of the caloric energy in our diet. Since fat is energy dense, providing 9 calories per gram, it is almost too easy to consume adequate amounts of energy each day through the consumption of dietary fat. Fat has fallen victim to the good versus bad mentality, which can often cloud the redeeming qualities that fat contributes to our overall health.

Fatty acids are to fats what saccharides are to carbohydrates and amino acids are to proteins. The main lipids in foods and in the body are triglycerides. Most triglycerides contain more than one type of fatty acid. Just like saccharides, fatty acids vary in the length of their carbon chains. The terms "saturated" and "unsaturated" refer to the number and location of single or double bonds with hydrogen on their carbon chain. Those that are fully loaded with single bonds to hydrogen are considered saturated fats. Saturated fats are typically solid at room temperature. Butter, lard, and even tropical oils like coconut oil in a cooler kitchen will all be solid, as they contain saturated fats. Fatty acid chains that are missing hydrogen and thus have double carbon bonds are called unsaturated fats. These fats are either monounsaturated or polyunsaturated, depending on the number of double bonds in the chain. In oil form, unsaturated fats will remain liquid at room temperature. Sources include nuts, seeds, avocados, olive oil, canola oil, peanut oil, tofu, soybeans, soybean oil, and corn oil. The level of saturation of a fatty acid will impact its physical features and storage capabilities.

You may be familiar with the term "hydrogenation," a process that converts polyunsaturated fats to saturated fats. This manufacturing process is intended to protect the fats from oxidation, which would have caused the fats to go stale and even rancid. The result also alters the texture and will make a normally liquid fat more solid at room temperature. This process, however, creates trans-fatty acids that damage health and are associated with increased risk for coronary heart disease, cancer, type 2 diabetes, and allergies. Major sources of trans fats in the SAD include margarine, shortening, commercial frying fats, high-fat baked goods, and salty snacks made with these fats. In my opinion, if you see the terms "hydrogenated" or "partially hydrogenated" anywhere on a food's packaging, do yourself a favor and place that food back where you found it and quickly walk in the opposite direction.

We store fat in adipose cells. The body's ability to do so as well as use large amounts of fat, as we cannot store large amounts of glycogen, allows us to survive without food for sustained periods of time—weeks and even months. Body fat also provides some other job duties that sometimes go unnoticed. Areas of structural fat throughout the body protect bones from pressure and hold organs and nerves in position, while also providing some cushioning to protect them from injury. Fat is an insulator, containing body heat and sustaining body temperature. Lipids are a necessary component of cellular structures, like the myelin sheath, which protects and insulates the cells of our central nervous system.

Dietary fat is certainly a multitasker. Fat is crucial for the proper digestion, absorption, and transport of fat-soluble vitamins and nutrients such as the carotenoids and lycopenes. The presence of dietary fat slows the digestive process down a bit by reducing gastric secretions, delaying gastric emptying, and promoting biliary and pancreatic secretions, which are necessary for proper digestion. Have you ever noticed that you're fuller longer after eating a meal or snack that contained fat?

We covered the essential amino acids when discussing proteins. There is also a class of essential fatty acids. They are the groups of fatty acids categorized as omega-6 and omega-3 fatty acids. You may be familiar with omega-3 fatty acids from fish oils or from plant-based options like nut and seed oils. These fatty acids have anti-inflammatory properties and have been shown to have beneficial effects in a variety of disease states, such as improved brain function during aging and cardiovascular disease. On the other hand, the Standard American Diet (SAD) is unfortunately far richer in omega-6 fatty acids than it is in omega-3, and ingesting both types of these fatty acids is pivotal for our health. This imbalance between the two essential fatty acids contributes to numerous diseases such as cardiovascular disease and depression, and chronic health issues like obesity, chronic inflammation, and immune issues that plague our population.

One of the major factors influencing this imbalance over the past thirty-plus years is the focus on low-fat diets. While the overall fat intake may have decreased, the consumption of proinflammatory omega-6 fats has sharply increased. As a result of this shift, Americans have consumed fewer anti-inflammatory, healthy omega-3s. In all of our sugar-fueled fat shaming, we've isolated the fats that provided the best armament against the effects of inflammation on metabolic dysfunction and excess fat tissue formation. Seems like a pretty cruel irony when you take a look at the science and how nutrition dogma steered so many down the wrong path. The optimal ratio of omega-6 to omega-3 fatty acids in the diet is 1:1 to 5:1. Being that we are currently around the 20:1 mark, we have a lot of work to do!

A CRUISE AROUND THE MICRONUTRIENTS

No discussion of basic nutrition is complete without briefly touching upon the micronutrients, as without them literally thousands of reactions and processes within the body would not occur properly, especially the processes we are most concerned with in terms of detoxification. Our nutrient needs vary and can be impacted by many factors like lifestyle, medications, genetics, etc. That said, there's no time like the present for members of the 50+ club to take an honest look at their intakes. If you have been consuming too much sugar or the SAD, chances are your diet has not provided you with sufficient amounts of vitamins and minerals. That, in turn, sets up some roadblocks on the detoxification superhighway. We'll take a deeper dive into the nutrient-driven pathways of detoxing later on.

A QUICK GLANCE AT THE MICRONUTRIENTS

- The body needs them in smaller amounts.
- They are not created by the body on its own in adequate amounts and, therefore, must be consumed.
- Insufficient intakes will cause health issues and deficiency syndromes.
- Vitamins are classified as either water-soluble or fat-soluble.
- Water-soluble vitamins include ascorbic acid (vitamin C) and the B vitamins—thiamin, riboflavin, niacin, vitamin B6 (pyridoxine, pyridoxal, and pyridoxamine), folacin, vitamin B12, biotin, and pantothenic acid.
- Fat-soluble vitamins include vitamins A, D, E, and K.
- Other micronutrients include macrominerals, trace minerals, and water.

WATER-SOLUBLE VITAMINS

Water-soluble vitamins dissolve in water. There is limited storage for them in the body. Water-soluble vitamins must be absorbed, and absorption can be impacted by source and quality of the nutrient, preparation methods, and the presence or absence of digestive issues.

Vitamin B1/Thiamine

- Necessary for energy metabolism and carbohydrate conversion. Plays a role in nerve and muscle activity. Additionally, B1 is linked to digestion and involvement with the health of skin, hair, eyes, mouth, liver, and the immune system.

- *Sources:* pork, organ meats, beans, peas, whole grains, brown rice, wheat germ, bran, brewer's yeast, blackstrap molasses, nuts, and sunflower seeds

Vitamin B2/Riboflavin

- Acts as a coenzyme in energy metabolism and carbohydrate conversion (coenzymes or cofactors are compounds that are necessary for an enzyme to do its job). It is involved in growth and development and red blood cell formation.

- Those at potential risk for a deficiency of B2 include those following a vegan/vegetarian diet or dairy-free diet, athletes, pregnant and lactating women, and infants.

- *Sources:* brewer's yeast, almonds, meats, organ meats, whole grains, wheat germ, mushrooms, soy, dairy, eggs, spinach, and oysters

Vitamin B3/Niacin

- Needed in cholesterol production, conversion of food into energy, digestion, and nervous system function. Niacin can be manufactured by the body from tryptophan.

- *Sources:* beans, beets, brewer's yeast, meats, poultry, organ meats, fish, seeds, nuts, and whole grains

Vitamin B5/Pantothenic Acid

- Needed in the conversion of food into energy, fat metabolism, sex and stress-related hormone production, nervous system function, red blood cell formation, immune function, and healthy digestion. Aids the body in using other nutrients.

- *Sources:* meats, vegetables, whole grains, legumes, lentils, egg yolks, milk, sweet potatoes, seeds, nuts, wheat germ, and salmon

Vitamin B6/Pyridoxine

- Involved in immune and nervous system function; protein, carbohydrate, and fat metabolism; and red blood cell production. Works with the synthesis of DNA/RNA and B12 absorption. B6 is essential in reducing homocysteine. Having an elevated homocysteine level is a risk factor for cardiac disease and is often associated with low levels of B vitamins, particularly B6, B12, and folate. It can also be caused by kidney issues, psoriasis, decreased thyroid hormone, and certain medications.

- *Sources:* poultry, tuna, salmon, shrimp, beef liver, lentils, soybeans, chickpeas, seeds, nuts, avocados, bananas, carrots, brown rice, bran, wheat germ, and whole grain flour

Vitamin B7/Biotin

- Plays a role in energy storage and protein, carbohydrate, and fat metabolism.

- It is synthesized by microbes in the gut.

- *Sources:* salmon, liver, pork, avocados, cauliflower, raspberries, whole grains, legumes, lentils, egg yolks, milk, sweet potatoes, seeds, nuts, and wheat germ

Vitamin B9/Folate

- A nutrient with a history of inadequate intakes, especially for women of childbearing age. Important for mental health and prevention of birth defects in infant DNA/RNA. Partners with B12 to regulate red blood cell production and iron function. Also reduces homocysteine.

- *Sources:* asparagus, avocados, fortified grains, tomato juice, green leafy vegetables, black-eyed peas, lentils, beans, and orange juice

Vitamin B12/Cobalamin

- Involved in the conversion of food into energy, nervous system function, red blood cell formation, iron function, and DNA/RNA synthesis. May be a nutrient lacking in the following situations: a poorly planned vegan/vegetarian diet, those with low stomach acid, and those on long-term proton pump inhibitor (PPI) medication.

- *Sources:* fish and seafood, meats, poultry, eggs, dairy products, and fortified cereals

Vitamin C/Ascorbic Acid

- A potent antioxidant, involved in collagen and tissue formation, wound healing, immune function, enzyme activation, transmitting hormonal information, blood clotting, cell and cell organelle membrane function, nerve impulse transmission, and muscular contraction and tone. Prevents weakness and irritability.

- *Sources:* broccoli, Brussels sprouts, cantaloupe, cauliflower, citrus, guava, kiwi, papaya, parsley, peas, potatoes, peppers, parsley, rose hips, strawberries, and tomatoes

FAT-SOLUBLE VITAMINS

These require the presence of fat in order to be dissolved in preparation for absorption. In contrast to water-soluble vitamins, extras of fat-soluble vitamins are stored in the liver and fat tissue, and they are usually not destroyed by cooking methods.

Vitamin A

- Essential for vision, immune function, skin and bone formation, cell growth and development, reproduction, gene regulation, and red blood cell formation.

- *Sources:* dairy, eggs, liver, fortified cereals, carrots, cantaloupe, green leafy vegetables, fruits, pumpkin, red peppers, and sweet potatoes

Vitamin D

- Necessary to maintain normal blood levels of calcium and phosphate, which is required for normal bone mineralization, muscle contraction, nerve conduction, and general cellular function in all of the body's cells. Vitamin D also impacts hormone and neurotransmitter production, immune function, and blood pressure regulation. Vitamin D is listed as a nutrient of concern for all age groups due to the prevalence of clinical deficiencies and insufficiencies; it is also a concern for those on long-term PPI medications, which can be a commonly used class of drug in the over-fifty crowd.

- *Sources:* sunlight, fortified dairy products, fish liver oil, fortified cereals, fortified orange juice, egg yolks, liver, fish, and fortified soy beverages

Vitamin E

- A potent antioxidant that regulates oxidation reactions, stabilizes cell membranes, aids in the formation of blood vessels, helps with immune function, and protects against cardiovascular disease, cataracts, and macular degeneration.

- *Sources:* wheat germ, liver, eggs, nuts, seeds, cold-pressed vegetable oils, dark leafy greens, sweet potatoes, avocados, asparagus, peanuts, peanut butter, and fortified cereals and juices

Vitamin K

- Works in blood clotting and calcium metabolism. Also aids the formation of glucose into glycogen for storage in the liver.

- *Sources:* green vegetables like kale, turnip greens, spinach, broccoli, lettuce, cabbage, beef liver, asparagus, watercress, cheese, oats, peas, whole wheat, and green tea

MACROMINERALS

Calcium

- Plays a role in blood clotting, bone and teeth formation, blood vessel constriction and relaxation, hormone secretion, nervous system function, and synergy with other nutrients to function. Currently a nutrient of concern for most due to inadequate intakes and long-term proton pump inhibitor medications.

- *Sources:* dairy, dairy alternative milks, wheat and soy flour, molasses, tofu, brewer's yeast, Brazil nuts, broccoli, cabbage, dark leafy greens, hazelnuts, oysters, sardines, and canned salmon

Phosphorus

- Involved with acid-base balance, hormone activation, bone formation, and energy production and storage.

- *Sources:* whole grains, enriched and fortified grain products, seafood, poultry, nuts, seeds, beans, peas, dairy, and meats

Magnesium

- Participates in over three hundred biochemical reactions that regulate muscle function, nerve function, heart rhythm, the immune system, and the development of strong bones. Regulates calcium, copper, zinc, potassium, and vitamin D.

- Magnesium is a nutrient of concern for all age groups as a result of increased intake of refined and processed foods, water softening systems, high alcohol consumption, gastrointestinal disorders, and certain medications that cause malabsorption. Insufficient magnesium intake poses a higher risk of metabolic syndrome, type 2 diabetes, cardiovascular disease, skeletal disorders, chronic obstructive pulmonary disease, depression, decreased cognition, and vitamin D deficiency.

- When consuming calcium or calcium supplements, be sure to include adequate magnesium. The optimal ratio of calcium to magnesium is 2 to 2.5. This is particularly important for the 50+ crowd as calcium's role in bone, breast, and cardiovascular health is often a topic of concern.

- *Sources:* avocados, bananas, beans and peas, green leafy vegetables, dairy products, nuts and pumpkin seeds, raisins, whole grains, potatoes, and wheat bran

Potassium

- Contributes to blood pressure regulation, fluid balance, growth and development, carbohydrate metabolism, heart function, muscle contraction, protein formation, and nervous system function. The SAD has caused potassium to be flagged as a nutrient of concern due to inadequate intakes; most Americans are only getting 54 percent of the recommended intake.

- *Sources:* dairy products, bananas, beans, tomatoes, spinach, prunes, sweet and white potatoes, oranges and orange juice, and beet greens

Sodium

- Involved with acid-base balance, fluid balance, muscle contraction, blood pressure regulation, and nervous system function. Flagged as a nutrient commonly consumed in excess as compared to the other electrolytes (potassium, magnesium, chloride, calcium, and phosphorus).

- *Sources:* table salt, poultry, baked goods, cheese, deli items, cured meats, snack foods, packaged/convenience/canned foods, soups (you may notice that many foods that are sources of sodium are not the most supportive of health and wellness)

Chloride

- Duties include acid-base balance, conversion of food into energy, fluid balance, digestion, and nervous system function.

- *Sources:* celery, lettuce, olives, rye, salt substitutes, seaweeds (e.g., dulse and kelp), tomatoes, table salt, and sea salt

TRACE MINERALS

Iron

- Continues to be recognized as an essential nutrient.

- Involved with energy production, immune function, red blood cell formation, and wound healing.

- Iron deficiency anemia unfortunately remains common despite the availability of iron-rich foods. It is important to have one's iron status evaluated not only to identify an anemia but also as excessive iron intake is linked to coronary heart disease and cancer.

- Can also be of concern with poorly planned vegan/vegetarian diets.
- *Sources:* beans and peas, dark green vegetables, enriched and fortified cereals and breads, meats, poultry, prunes and prune juice, raisins, seafood, and whole grains

Chromium

- Assists insulin function and involved in carbohydrate and fat metabolism. It may also have a beneficial effect on serum triglyceride levels and regulation of gene expression.
- *Sources:* brewer's yeast, whole grains, seafood, green beans, broccoli, prunes, nuts, potatoes, meats, spices (e.g., garlic and cinnamon), basil, turkey, apples, bananas, and grape and orange juices

Copper

- An antioxidant involved in bone formation, collagen and connective tissue formation, energy production, hair and skin coloring, and taste sensitivity. Stimulates iron absorption and nervous system function; helps metabolize several fatty acids.
- *Sources:* oysters, seeds, dark leafy vegetables, organ meats, dried legumes, whole grains, nuts, shellfish, lentils, chocolate, cocoa, soybeans, oats, and blackstrap molasses

Zinc

- Supports over three hundred enzymes, the immune system, wound healing, taste/smell, bone mass health, DNA synthesis, and the expression of genetic information.
- *Sources:* oysters, red meat, poultry, beans, nuts, seafood, whole grains, fortified breakfast cereals, and dairy

Manganese

- Plays an essential role in carbohydrate, protein, fat, and cholesterol metabolism; cartilage and bone formation; and wound healing.

- *Sources:* beans, nuts, pineapple, spinach, sweet potato, and whole grains

Molybdenum

- Involved with enzyme production.

- *Sources:* beans and peas, nuts, and whole grains

Iodine

- Needed for metabolism and thyroid hormone production.

- *Sources:* breads and cereals, dairy products, iodized salt, potatoes, seafood, seaweed, and turkey

Selenium

- An antioxidant that works with vitamin E and helps with immune function and prostaglandin production.

- *Sources:* brewer's yeast, wheat germ, liver, butter, cold-water fish, shellfish, garlic, whole grains, sunflower seeds, and Brazil nuts

WATER

Ah, the fluid of life. Remember the survival phrase, "You can go three weeks without food, three days without water, and only three minutes without air"? Water is essential to life and also to a body in balance. Roughly 60 percent of an adult's body weight is from water. Comparing body composition values, lean muscle is made up of about 75 percent water and fat tissue 25 percent. Besides its obvious role of keeping you hydrated, water is also an essential transportation system, carrying nutrients while removing waste products and acting as a cushion, a solvent, and even a lubricant. Water is vital to maintaining blood volume and the structural integrity of large molecules within the body. It is a multitasker that's also a necessary component of numerous metabolic reactions and maintaining balance in regulating your body temperature. With an inadequate intake of water, your physical as well as mental sharpness and performance will be negatively impacted. Major organ systems of the body also rely heavily upon hydration to continue functioning properly.

If you wait until you feel thirsty before you decide to hydrate with water, you are already way behind the eight ball since the body is already dehydrated by the time thirst mechanisms are triggered. This process also becomes dulled as we age, thus making older adults and the elderly at even greater risk for dehydration. You may have grown up with the phrase, "Drink eight 8-ounce glasses of water every day." Some conventional nutrition wisdom is not entirely off base; however, a simple rule of thumb is to be sure that you are drinking half of your body weight in ounces each day. Please note, if you are obese, using an ideal or adjusted body weight to determine a fluid ounce goal is appropriate. Be sure to take into consideration any additional fluid losses that may occur through exercise and even during illness. It will be especially important during your sugar detox that you are mindful of your hydration status and are diligent about getting enough fluids each and every day.

Common signs of dehydration, besides the obvious thirst sensation, include fatigue, dry mouth, muscle weakness, flushing of the skin, decreased urine output, and even mood changes such as increased apathy and impatience. These symptoms will only worsen as the state of dehydration worsens. Be certain to look out for difficulties with focusing or concentrating, headaches, insomnia, worsening irritability, rapid breathing, and changes in body temperature. These are all signs of deepening dehydration. Once severe dehydration sets in, symptoms include muscle spasms, loss of balance and coordination, delirium, exhaustion, dizziness, and even collapse.

Now that we've covered some of the basic nutrients, we can move on to discussing how we can make them work in your favor.

CHAPTER 2

AN AMERICAN HORROR STORY: THE STANDARD AMERICAN DIET

Have you ever asked yourself why there are so many diet books out there? It seems as if a new one hits the shelves every day. People's dietary habits are personal and driven by many different things. Take a moment to reflect now on the influences that drive your dietary choices. They could be emotional, social, religious, cultural, and economical. As we explore some basic dietary guidelines in this chapter, I want to consider how your choices have been stacking up and where the voids are. Diet books may seem like a dime a dozen, with new ones being published almost daily. Why is it that the market for diet info never becomes saturated? Maybe the reason for that is to illustrate how there is no one-size-fits-all approach. Personally, I don't believe in a one-size-fits-most approach. I believe in practicing personalized nutrition with my clients.

Here, my goal is to help you identify some of the root causes and influences on your diet, as well as to help you identify some of the reasons why you are gravitating toward more sugar-laden, highly processed, refined carbohydrate–based foods. If you're like most of us, chances are you've probably tried multiple diets throughout your lifetime. You may also have achieved a degree of success with one or more of them. The question is, how sustainable was the success?

How many times have you been on a rapid weight-loss roller coaster with a variety of crash diets that failed to yield long-term success and contributed to a vicious cycle of yo-yo dieting while potentially wreaking havoc on your metabolism in the process? There is certainly a body of evidence to support almost any and every single style of diet out there if you look hard enough. The tipping point is the quality of the evidence.

Sadly, even though there was a lack of quality, unbiased, evidence-based research proving that a low-fat diet was the cure-all for our nation's rising rates of obesity, diabetes, and heart disease, it became the adopted nutritional standard across the land. Food manufacturers do a wonderful job of reacting quickly to changing tastes, preferences, and popular diet trends. The low-fat diet craze was definitely no exception. Before long, entire lines of products touted as low fat, reduced fat, and fat free or cholesterol free were readily available. Fat provides flavor and texture. When a manufacturer has to reformulate a product to remove or reduce fat, flavor and texture suffer. In order to make a product remain palatable and, more importantly, marketable, fats and cholesterol were soon replaced with various forms of sugar and processed carbohydrates. Remember those green boxes of SnackWell's cookies that were all the rage in the early 1990s, at the height of the fat-free craze? People were devouring boxes of these cookies thinking they were a guilt-free, healthy choice because they were fat free. It was a perfect example of clever marketing combined with nutritional misinformation, as these cookies still contained just as much sugar as their unaltered competitors.

Needless to say, butter and healthy fats were ousted from our diets, and sugar, starches, and fake fats reigned supreme. With the combination of the fat-free diet and the Food Guide Pyramid being preached all across the land as the gospel of the healthy American diet, there now existed a perfect storm ready to unleash years of nutritional collateral damage and exponentially high health-care costs.

Believe me, I was raised in the midst of this paradigm shift in nutritional teachings and even had it hammered into my head during my undergraduate dietetics program. I thought I had to be doing something wrong. I counted calories, points, grams of fat, the whole gamut, but I was always hungry regardless of how much "healthy" food I ate within my "allowances." I couldn't sustain weight loss and was living proof of a flawed program, struggling for years with my weight. While learning the hard way, I often asked my patients if they knew what the definition of insanity is: doing the same thing over and over again and expecting a different response.

IS FAT A LOADED GUN?

A major issue of the low-fat craze is it threw all fats under the bus. When it came to dietary fats, the baby was tossed out with the bathwater. Yes, saturated fats, which occur mostly in animal products, were part of the equation in the battle of the bulge, but they were not the sole enemy they were portrayed to be. Too little emphasis and education were placed on differentiating healthy fats from unhealthy fats. To this day, especially when evaluating the pros and cons of eating fats, there's a public knowledge deficit on how organic, grass-fed, pastured foods compare to conventional farmed and raised foodstuffs. For decades, we were conditioned to think that eating eggs, butter, cheese, and animal meats put us on the fast track to heart disease and a statin prescription because they would raise your blood fats, cholesterol, and triglycerides, a form of fats linked to arterial plaque formation as well as free radicals, which are known to cause damage to cells, DNA, and enzymes in the body. Healthier fats (that actually reduce cardiovascular risks), such as nuts, seeds, extra-virgin olive oil, and essential omega-3 fats from cold-water fish were also lumped into this category.

Since this book is titled *The Sugar Detox Diet for 50+*, my assumption is those who will be reading it will be aged fifty and over. That said, you've most likely been subjected to old-school nutritional dogma banishing and demonizing fats and proclaiming carbs as king. Now, don't misunderstand me. I'm not bashing carbohydrates either. What's missing from the conversation on carbohydrates, proteins, and fats has always been a lack of emphasis on the quality and source.

You may remember in 1972 when *The New Diet Revolution* by Dr. Atkins began stirring the pot and questioning the belief that the only way to successfully lose weight was through a diet rich in complex carbohydrates but restrictively low in fat. "Complex carbohydrates" was one of the key factors that got lost in translation, as most Americans were actually eating the Standard American Diet's refined, highly processed carbohydrates. As we approach the fifty-year mark since Dr. Atkins's book was first published, numerous books have been added to the Atkins line, along with many other books hopping on this topic's bandwagon. In 1996 came *Sugar Busters*, then in 2003, *The South Beach Diet Cookbook* and a revised *The New Sugar Busters*, just to name a few. For many die-hard conventional diet holdouts, it was an easier pill to swallow that eating fat makes you fat, when in actuality you should not blame the butter alone for what the bread was also doing to you.

So, let's examine this a little further. These lower-carb diets challenge the old nutritional tenet that the healthiest weight-management program is high in carbohydrates, adequate in protein, and low in fat. You may have followed one of these low-fat, higher-carbohydrate diets in the past or know people who did. They may even have gone so far as to virtually eliminate fat. Even with such extremes, many remained unsuccessful in their weight-loss efforts. Conventional nutritional wisdom of the 1990s encouraged the public to consume of six to eleven servings of grains per day—the largest portion of the Food Guide Pyramid. Stuck at the tippy top, the smallest portion of your dietary intake was to come from healthy fats and oils. You can imagine the backlash that Dr. Atkins and his constituents would have faced when literally trying to turn the pyramid on its head.

The lower-carb camp believed that consuming too many carbohydrates actually forces the body to convert the excess calories to fat, thus contributing to obesity, higher blood fat levels, and insulin resistance. In fact, from a metabolic standpoint, a high-carbohydrate diet can trigger elevated triglyceride levels. Referring back to our discussion on insulin and glucagon, when you consume high amounts of carbohydrates, you trigger the release of a large amount of insulin to respond to this whopping dose of glucose. When the system works as nature intended, insulin encourages the muscles to take in glucose and stimulates the synthesis of fat and glycogen. As a result, your blood glucose level would then return to a normal range. Intestinal absorption is usually completed within about two hours after a meal; however, the effects of insulin continue, which causes your blood glucose levels to fall. Your body, in turn, views this hypoglycemic state (low blood sugar level) as a state of starvation, triggering a release of countermeasures, again to obtain balance. Counterregulatory hormones stimulate the release of free fatty acids from fat cells in the body, which are then packed into transport lipoproteins in your liver, causing an increase in your blood triglyceride levels.

THE GLYCEMIC INDEX

Now that we're on the topic of insulin secretion, it's a good time for a brief discussion on the glycemic index. The glycemic index (GI), developed in the 1980s by Dr. David Jenkins, is a scale ranging from 0 to 100 that measures the rises in blood glucose and insulin triggered by a specific food.

The standard of comparison is to 50 grams of glucose, which has a GI of 100. If the glycemic index of a tested food is 50, then it was shown to raise blood sugar only 50 percent as fast as glucose does. Generally speaking, foods that have a GI of 55 or less are considered low glycemic, 56 to 69 is moderate, and 70 to 100 is high.

How is the GI of a food determined? Imagine that ten or more healthy people are fed a portion of a food containing 50 grams of digestible carbohydrates, and then the effect on their blood glucose levels is measured over the next two hours. On a separate day, the same ten people consume an equal-carbohydrate portion of the sugar glucose, which serves as the control point, and their two-hour blood glucose response is also measured. A GI value to the test food is then calculated for each person by dividing their glucose response to the test food by their glucose response to the control food. The final GI value for the test food is the average GI value for the ten people. Why does this matter? The more rapidly your blood sugar rises in response to a meal or snack, the quicker it will fall and, generally, it will fall lower than where it was prior to the meal. Carbohydrate foods with a low GI value (55 or less) are more slowly digested, absorbed, and metabolized, thereby causing a lower and slower rise in blood glucose and, therefore, corresponding insulin levels. Most fruits and vegetables, beans, minimally processed grains, pasta, dairy foods, and nuts will have a low GI value. Most of your carbohydrate choices should ideally be lower in GI value. Moderate GI foods include white and sweet potatoes, corn, brown rice, couscous, and some breakfast cereals, including those promoted as healthy, like cream of wheat and shredded wheat. So go easy on this group. High-GI foods to avoid are white bread, rice cakes, most crackers, bagels, cakes, doughnuts, croissants, and most packaged breakfast cereals—even instant oatmeal and cornflakes.

How many of your current food choices fall into the moderate or high categories? Remember, foods that are considered high on the glycemic index can trigger the reward and food craving areas of the brain, as seen with other addictions. These foods generally result in a rapid rise in blood sugar and, ultimately, a rapid fall in blood sugar called rebound hypoglycemia, which is a result of the action of insulin. This sharp decrease in blood sugar levels can cause cravings for more food, especially high-GI foods. These cravings and hunger signals are fueled by the changes in your blood sugar levels. Furthermore, you will typically begin experiencing hunger sensations sooner than you would have if your last meal or snack had a more balanced macronutrient profile.

Have you ever heard the word "hangry" or seen the commercials for a certain candy bar teasing the viewer that they "aren't themselves when they're hungry" and thus need to eat the advertised candy bar? We've all experienced being hangry at one point in our lives, or being so hungry but we would eat the quickest thing we could get our hands on regardless of the healthfulness of that choice. During these episodes, we typically consume far more than necessary, especially of quick carbs, because the signaling messengers that tell the body and brain that blood sugar level has normalized is delayed.

Sadly, this spurs a vicious cycle into perpetual motion, one that greatly contributes to the roller-coaster ride of powerful cravings, headaches, anxiety, difficulty with focus and concentration, sleeplessness, and fatigue. It also leads to increased insulin levels, inflammation, and elevated blood triglyceride levels. This pattern has created a wide-open door for obesity and diabetes.

GLYCEMIC LOAD

Expanding on the concept of the glycemic index, glycemic load (GL) provides a more accurate illustration of how the carbohydrates we consume impact blood sugar. It gives a more detailed picture than GI alone because GI only indicates how rapidly a particular carbohydrate turns into sugar, while GL indicates the amount of carbohydrate in a serving, thereby taking into consideration both the quality and quantity of carbohydrate in one measurement. Glycemic load, not glycemic index, better predicts blood glucose values of different types and amounts of food. The formula to calculate GL is GL = (GI x the amount of carbohydrate) divided by 100.

As new products are continually hitting the market, any reference books on the GI/GL are usually obsolete before they even hit bookshelves. I generally discourage my clients from getting too wrapped up in numbers. This can be a doorway to more stress and, ultimately, more imbalanced choices.

The path of least resistance to stay in line with a lower-GI diet is to choose the foods we discussed that fall into the low-GI category. The recipes in this book will all be low-GI as well. If you're craving more info on GI, the Aussies are ahead of the curve here, so for the most comprehensive resources, check out the University of Sydney's GI website at http://www.glycemicindex.com and the Glycemic Index Foundation's site at https://www.gisymbol.com.

SUGAR ON THE CHOPPING BLOCK?

Why, now, is sugar and not fat currently on the chopping block of what to remove from your diet? There is no denying that the shift in food choices toward simple carbs and sugary processed foods has greatly contributed to the escalation in rates of chronic disease such as type 2 diabetes, cardiovascular disease, and, of course, obesity.

Why have we seen such a dramatic shift in the American palate? Factors include increased stress in daily life, socioeconomic issues, lack of access to quality health care, and unequal access to quality food. Populations that have been most impacted are those with lower socioeconomic status, women, and children. Research shows immigrants within one generation's time living in the US shift to acculturate to the Standard American Diet, trading their traditional and indigenous food preferences for animal products and processed, packaged convenience foods with higher amounts of sugars, poor-quality fats, oils, and carbohydrates.

But it's not just low-income populations that are experiencing dietary pattern changes. The middle and upper classes are also impacted by supersized portions and increased frequencies of snacking and dining out. Lest we forget the latter factor, how many calories are you consuming per day from sweetened beverages? According to the NIH, from the late 1970s to the mid-1990s, calories provided from milk consumption decreased by 38 percent while those provided from sugar-sweetened drinks jumped up 135 percent.

LUST FOR QUICK FIXES

Truth is, the carbohydrates that we typically eat today are not our grandmothers' carbohydrates. We have stripped the grains naked, removing most if not all of the fiber as well as the micronutrients. Today, Americans are eating far more foods made from white flours, and in much larger portions, than in previous generations. Just look at the difference in size between a muffin served in the 1950s or 1960s and the giant muffins served today (and typically consumed in one sitting, to boot). We've swapped out whole grain hot cereals and whole grain breakfast breads for instant oats, processed breakfast cereals, and breakfast cookies that masquerade as healthy choices.

In our quest for all things quick and easy, we've even stripped and processed something as basic as rice. As a result of our lust for quick fixes, we have sacrificed nutrition and created an entire category of calorically dense yet nutritionally deficient foods. We load up on these deficient foods and then expect our bodies to perform optimally. I can't think of a more prime example of setting oneself up for failure by way of fuel choice. Adding insult to injury, we've been programmed to believe that a big bowl of cold cereal is the best way to start off the day. Well, if you're choosing one of the majority of commercial cereals on the market and topping it with fat-phobic skim or 1 percent milk, you are beginning your day with an out-of-balance, high-carbohydrate, lower-protein, low-fat meal that will set your blood sugar roller coaster in motion for the day.

As we continue to explore our keyword "balance," one constant will be to bring the macronutrient composition of our meals and snacks into balance in order to prevent even getting on the roller coaster at all.

Further fueling our dependence on quick, easy, but highly processed foods is the change to our lifestyle habits, like the withering away of family dinners at home. As a result of the move to consuming more and more meals prepared outside of our homes, our caloric intake has almost doubled while the quality has declined.

Pause for a moment here to think about the following:

- How many meals per week do you eat outside of your home?
- How many meals per week do you eat prepared by your own hand or a family member's?
- How much time per day do you spend on cooking and preparing food?

The 2014 Eating & Health Module study, which is part of the Bureau of Labor Statistics' American Time Use Survey, illustrated that the average American spent only thirty minutes or so per day on meal preparation and cleanup. That should speak volumes. If you're spending more time than that each day, consider yourself ahead of the curve. But if it is not much more, then there's probably some room for improvement. If you're in the thirty-and-under camp, then looking at ways to incorporate more meal planning and preparation will be a valuable asset to success in cutting out sugar and maintaining a healthy diet over the long term.

Cherry-picked, sponsored research conducted by industry with strong lobbyists and deep pockets clouds the data on healthy food choices even further for the average layperson. This type of sponsored research only serves to undermine more ethical research aimed at providing an unbiased recommendation on minimum and maximum suggested intakes, not only for sugar and carbohydrates but also for animal proteins such as meats, dairy, and eggs.

CURRENT DIET GUIDELINES

Thankfully, science is catching up to those of us in the functional nutrition camp. It's beginning to recognize that labeling nutrients as either good or bad does little to yield positive outcomes. You may or may not be aware of the gradual shift in the USDA's Dietary Guidelines for Americans. The USDA began issuing dietary recommendations as early as 1894, and the first USDA food guide, *Food for Young Children*, was released in 1916. In 1980, the first edition of *Nutrition and Your Health: Dietary Guidelines for Americans* was published. The focus was on a variety of foods, not quantities, and included recommendations on maintaining a healthy body weight and moderating one's consumption of fat, saturated fat, cholesterol, and sodium. Since 1980, the *Dietary Guidelines for Americans* have been revised and republished every five years.

In fact, the dietary guidelines advisory committee that formulated the 2015–2020 Dietary Guidelines (see the Addendum on page 242 for an update regarding the 2020–2025 guidelines) concluded that low-fat diets did not have a beneficial effect on cardiovascular disease. Thereafter, the recommendation shifted toward the inclusion of healthful fats.

The 2015–2020 Dietary Guidelines for Americans are:

- Follow a healthy eating pattern across the lifespan.
- Focus on a variety of nutrient-dense foods and the amount of food being consumed.
- Limit calories from added sugars and saturated fats, and reduce sodium.
- Shift to healthier food and beverage choices.
- Support a healthy eating pattern for all.

One goal of the 2015–2020 Dietary Guidelines is to provide the information Americans need to make healthy food choices. The current guidelines are based on the above five umbrella guidelines, which we'll spend some time examining in relation to our sugar detox goals.

GUIDELINE 1: FOLLOW A HEALTHY EATING PATTERN ACROSS THE LIFESPAN

This focuses on looking at the big picture of how your dietary choices add up/measure up over your lifetime. Consider your current eating habits and patterns, for they have a significant impact on your health. Over the course of this book, we're going to be looking at how to improve your eating habits and dietary patterns because food truly is medicine and can be one of your most powerful resources in disease management and prevention.

GUIDELINE 2: FOCUS ON VARIETY, NUTRIENT DENSITY, AND AMOUNT

Personally, I think one important word—"quality"—is omitted from guideline #2. We can assume that that would be an unwritten component of nutrient density; however, we all know what happens when we assume. The main takeaway for this guideline is to focus more on ensuring that your healthy eating pattern keeps you within the appropriate number of calories based on your age, gender, and level of activity while also meeting your nutritional needs in a sustainable and realistic manner.

One key concept very relevant to our sugar detox goals is nutrient density. Back to the balance equation: nutrient-dense foods provide the right balance. They're packed full of the nutrients we need to thrive but without the addition of poor-quality fats, sugars, refined starches, or sodium. Essentially, nutrient-dense foods build the foundation for a healthy diet.

My suggested examples of nutrient-dense foods to build the foundation of a long-term, realistic, balanced diet:

- Choose a variety of vegetables. Include all the colors of the rainbow: dark green, blue, purple, yellow, red, and orange.
- Include more plant-based proteins: nuts, seeds, legumes (beans and peas).
- Go easy with starchy vegetables.

- Eat your fruits, especially whole fruits, and try not to drink them. Consume more vegetables than fruits.

- If consuming grains, make sure that at least half of them are whole grains.

- If consuming dairy, including milk, yogurt, and cheese, opt for organic, grass-fed reduced-fat or full-fat products, with no artificial sweeteners.

- If consuming animal protein, aim for wild-caught seafood, organic grass-fed lean meats, poultry, and eggs.

- Choose minimally processed, cold-pressed, organic, and preferably virgin or extra-virgin oils.

(I'll have more extensive food lists for you later in the book.)

GUIDELINE 3: LIMIT CALORIES FROM ADDED SUGARS AND SATURATED FATS; REDUCE SODIUM INTAKE

Finally, the Dietary Guidelines took a stance with some specific suggested limits.

Added Sugars: Limit to less than 10 percent of total calories daily.

The natural sugars in fruits, vegetables, and milk are not added sugars. We'll chat more about them later too. The confusion over sugars and carbs is also contributing to revisions of the nutrition facts labeling. It is now easier to read the actual carbohydrate breakdown of a food item by total carbs, added sugars, and fiber. Of course, if you're choosing items that do not require packaging and a nutrition facts label, then you greatly reduce your risk of consuming added sugars.

I want to drive home the following fact: Added sugars add calories without providing any other nutritional value. There is no way for someone to claim they have a healthy eating pattern when their diet is high in added sugars. Evaluating where your sources of added sugars are coming from is an important step in moving toward detoxing from them. The most common culprit is beverages: more than 50 percent of added sugar intake comes from what we choose to drink, such as juices, soft drinks, and energy drinks.

Fats: Limit saturated fats to less than 10 percent of total calories daily, and limit trans fats to as low as possible (preferably zero for trans fats, in my opinion).

This is one area where the debate surrounding fat still rages, as there is a significant difference between the fat profiles of poor-quality, processed oils and organic, cold-pressed oils as well as between conventionally raised animal fats and organic, grass-fed, pastured animal fats. Yes, research has shown that diets high in saturated (from conventionally produced sources) and trans fats are associated with heart disease. This is one of the main reasons why foods high in saturated fats like butter, whole milk, and meats have been under attack for decades, prompting the low-fat/fat-free movement and the slew of problematic products that accompanied the war on fat.

Avoid trans fats, hands down, at all costs. The main sources are processed foods, like desserts, frozen pizza, and coffee creamer. Remember, if you see the words "hydrogenated" or "partially hydrogenated" anywhere on the food label of a product you are considering putting into your body, you can be guaranteed it's a source of trans fats. One little tidbit about our current food labeling laws is that if a serving of a product contains 0.5 grams or less of trans fat, the manufacturer has the option to list the amount of trans fat on the label as zero. Now, ask yourself the last time you picked up a bag of snack chips with a 1-ounce serving size. Did you only consume 1 ounce in a sitting? If you're like most people, the answer is probably no. So, let's say for the sake of argument, you consumed the entire bag of chips cooked in hydrogenated or partially hydrogenated oils from the Kwik-E-Mart that was labeled to contain three servings and 0 trans fat (even if it did contain 0.5 grams per serving). You have potentially now consumed 1.5 grams of trans fat from those chips and exceeded the recommended limit. Play it safe and back away from any item with the words "hydrogenated" or "partially hydrogenated" on the label. Your body will thank you for that choice.

Sodium: Limit to less than 2,300 milligrams daily (for adults and children fourteen years and older)

It's no secret that many Americans get 50 percent more sodium than what is recommended and that high sodium intakes are often associated with high blood pressure and heart disease. Diets high in sodium typically lack other important electrolyte nutrients such as magnesium, potassium, calcium, phosphate, and chloride.

Alcohol: Limit to no more than one drink daily for women and no more than two for men.

Simple fact here is if you currently do not drink, do not start drinking alcohol for any "perceived" health reason, and evaluate possible reasons why you shouldn't drink, such as contraindication with certain medications, medical diagnoses, or during pregnancy (just because one may be over fifty doesn't entirely rule out the pregnancy possibility, I've seen many exceptions to rules in my twenty-five-plus years of practice!).

GUIDELINE 4: SHIFT TO HEALTHIER FOOD AND BEVERAGE CHOICES

Small, gradual, realistic changes can reap big rewards and be more sustainable over time. Even amid our discussion of shifting away from sugar and of sugar detoxing, the ultimate goal is for long-lasting diet and lifestyle change.

GUIDELINE 5: SUPPORT HEALTHY EATING PATTERNS FOR ALL

Health and disease statistics clearly illustrate that the vast majority of Americans aren't following these dietary recommendations. Besides working on improving your own personal eating pattern, I challenge you to also pay it forward and consider how you can support others in improving their eating patterns. Some suggestions for you to consider include:

- Add more veggies to favorite dishes, and feature them more as an entrée rather than only as a "side dish."

- Plan meals as a family, and cook at home. Get everyone involved more with mealtime.

- Get moving. Incorporate physical activity into time with family or friends.

- Support healthier options in our schools and workplaces.

- Get involved with or even start a community garden or farmers market.

- Avoid the urge to dump your poorer-quality pantry items at food donation centers. You may mean well, but the fact of the matter is that underserved populations are at the highest risk of nutrient deficiencies. So, donate healthy foods to support shelters and food banks.

After reviewing your current diet, how are you stacking up against these guidelines? Are you on a SAD trajectory? Make mental notes of what has been working well in your diet and lifestyle, and where you require improvement.

FINDING BALANCE FOR LONG-TERM SUCCESS

Let's revisit our theme of balance. The downward spiral of imbalances initiated by the current American diet does not just shift total calories but impacts multiple domains in the ecology of the human body:

- carbohydrate quality
- dietary fiber intake
- electrolyte balance
- acid-base balance
- fatty acid balance

- micronutrient balance
- macronutrient balance
- phytonutrient balance
- glycemic balance
- insulin balance

Achieving balance is a primary goal for long-term success. While numerous styles of dieting are promoted today, balance and personalization are key. Short-term fixes rarely translate into long-term sustainable practices. Please don't let the title of this book or the fact that the term "detox" is included fool you into believing that this is going to be just another crash diet. Together, we will outline short-term as well as long-term changes to make in your food choices to bring balance and harmony to your health and wellness.

The Institute of Medicine (IOM) lists the recommended dietary intake for adults as 45–65 percent of daily calories from carbohydrates, 20–35 percent from fat, and 10–35 percent from protein. I consider these to be guidelines, certainly not gospel, and you may find that your body thrives with personal ratios on target with IOM's or slightly different. That's part of the beauty behind embarking on a wellness journey—the opportunity to silence the outside noise of all the other influences and truly be open to the signals your body is sending. Illness is your body screaming for attention. In order to achieve wellness you have to listen for the whispers, not just the screams.

Consider carbs and fats as fuel; protein is building materials. Now, think of your body as a physical structure. You need a balance of energy to build that structure, along with the materials required to build it with. But is it cost effective to burn your building materials as a fuel source? Absolutely not! We want adequate protein to maintain our building. The standard recommendation for protein intake is 0.8 to 1.0 grams per kilogram of body weight. For example, if you weighed 120 pounds, you would need only about 50 grams of protein. For most following the Standard American Diet, that would almost feel like a protein restriction. So, before we go any further, let's put to rest the diet claims that you need high amounts of protein to lose weight, or as part of cutting carbs, or to just be healthy. If anything, it's quite the opposite. Much of the emerging research on longevity, healthy aging, cancer, and other common chronic health issues has shown that diets high in protein can actually contribute to negative health outcomes. People who live in "blue zones," areas of the world that have the highest percentages of centenarians (people living to one hundred years or greater), actually consume a relatively low-protein diet.

Our shared goal with this book is not only to help you get off of sugar, but also to provide some tools for you to explore what combinations of macronutrients your body prefers. Each of us is a bio-individual, a unique combination of genes; therefore, a one-size-fits-all mentality does not apply when seeking person-alized nutrition goals. You may even find the other members of your household vary in what they consider optimal diets. Truth be told, my husband and I follow distinctively different styles of eating, but we each do what makes our bodies feel best. In working toward balance, it's important to remember that increasing your intake of one macronutrient can usually result in decreases of another. We are not aiming here to tip your macronutrient intake out of balance, but rather to rein in the imbalanced intakes of sugar. I raise this point merely to illustrate that with so many styles of diets being promoted these days, one can easily fall victim to triggering a potential imbalance and even nutrient insufficiencies if not being mindful of the nutrients provided by the macronutrient group being avoided or reduced.

There is absolutely nothing wrong with seeking out your body's preferences. Overall, a healthy eating pattern limits added sugars, ultra-processed foods, refined carbohydrates, poor-quality refined fats and oils, and poor-quality animal proteins.

QUALITY IS A CHOICE

I have mentioned a few times by now that quality trumps quantity. Let's explore that a bit further. First, I want you to ask yourself the following questions:

- Do I tend to be penny wise and dollar foolish?
- Do I believe in making an investment in my own health?
- Do I make my food choices based solely on cost?

One of the most common objections I hear from my clients is that eating healthy is "expensive." On the surface, that may appear to be true, and our "need it right now" society has made it cheaper to eat burgers and fries than a salad. We don't need to spend a lot of time reviewing the hundreds of studies linking poor dietary choices to negative health outcomes. Sadly, the studies supporting the numerous health benefits of choosing organic, grass-fed, non-genetically modified foods don't get nearly as much attention.

As you get closer to retirement, besides your typical investment portfolio, I challenge you to consider your health and wellness portfolio to be equally important. While I am not an investment broker or an economist, when it comes to shedding light on food choices, an economics analogy can be useful and motivating. Take the debate over choosing organic over nonorganic foods. The term "ROI" means return on investment. While choosing organic foods may result in a slightly higher grocery bill, consider it an investment in your health. You earn returns and gains through improved health and wellness. Even the stock market has highs and lows, and any broker will tell you that the best investments have long-term returns. Your weekly investment in organic foods will yield not only short-term rewards as you feel better, but also much greater rewards over the long haul. These include decreased risk for chronic, diet-related diseases, improvement in your quality of life, an increase in productivity, and a decreased need for doctor's visits and medications. Furthermore, with health-care costs being a concern for so many of us, common sense would be to opt for an investment plan that includes focusing on your food as part of your preventative prescriptive intervention. Imagine fewer copays and more money to play with in retirement, all while eating better-tasting foods. Sounds like a win-win to me!

If you're not yet entirely convinced to hop on the organic, non-GMO bandwagon, then at least reassess the quality of your food choices—today. Start out with your produce choices, as you'll be eating more of them as you move away from sugar. I often recommend and personally use the Environmental Working Group's Shopping Guides. They have a wonderful website and, yes, they even have an app. I encourage you to visit www.ewg.org and download the "Clean Fifteen" and "Dirty Dozen" lists now, and definitely as you prepare for your sugar detox. As the name implies, the Clean Fifteen lists the top fifteen produce items with the least amount of pesticides and residues in the edible portion. These are the produce items you do not necessarily need to buy organic. Conversely, the Dirty Dozen are the twelve produce items with the highest amounts of pesticides and residues. Thus, you certainly want to make the investment in buying organic for these. Check these lists every so often for updates and seasonal changes.

These small steps forward, along with breaking up with sugar, will be powerful investments in your health. Poor-quality foods to steer clear of include: highly processed snack foods, sugar-laden beverages, refined (white) grains, refined sugar, fried foods, foods high in saturated and trans fats, conventionally raised animal products, and high-glycemic foods. Get comfortable with reading labels. If a food has more than five ingredients, if sugar is in the first three ingredients, or if you can't pronounce the ingredients, it's most likely not going to be a healthy choice, so put it back on the shelf and walk away. Avoid Frankenfoods; if you need a chemistry set to create the food you are considering eating, DON'T eat it. Better yet, what would you choose to eat if I were dining with you? (Don't worry, my friends know that I'm not the food police.)

It may take some time, but your taste buds and your body will thank you as you begin to experience flavors beyond just sweet and salty. You will find a new appreciation for real, whole, minimally processed food. Real food is not only nourishing but also amazingly delicious. One of my favorite food quotes is, "You can't expect to feel like a million bucks when you're eating from the dollar menu!" Don't shortchange yourself! Food is not just calories, numbers, macros, and micros. Food is a bounty of information to our cells and serves to nourish us mind, body, and spirit.

CHOOSE A VARIETY

Remember, variety is the spice of life, and we need a variety of foods each and every day in our diet in order to obtain all of the nutrients that we need. Variety is even more important today than it was for our grandparents' generation as the foods they ate had a much higher nutrient content than what we typically eat today. Nutrient depletion in the soil combined with modern farming practices have led to significant declines in the levels of calcium, phosphorus, vitamin C, iron, and riboflavin, just to name a few, in our foods. If you needed a reason to opt for organic produce as much as possible, nutrient depletion alone should be motivation enough. Many Americans barely come close to recommended intakes of vegetables and fruits while being way over recommended intakes of added sugars, refined carbohydrates, and poor-quality fats and oils. (PS: If you want a great read on choosing the best varieties of produce based on those that have mostly closely retained their nutrient density profile over the generations, I recommend Jo Robinson's book *Eating on the Wild Side.*)

CHAPTER 3

FUELING UP THE BODY

In order to fuel the needs of the body and maintain life, we need a regular supply of energy. But after we eat a meal and digest the macronutrients, how does the energy get dispersed and how are fuel levels maintained?

UNDERSTANDING NUTRIENT METABOLISM

In Chapter 1, we discussed carbohydrate digestion. After digestion in the intestinal tract, glucose travels to the liver, where about 50 percent is converted to glycogen for storage in the liver and muscles. Because glycogen needs to be stored with water, it takes up a lot of space. Therefore, we only carry about sixteen to eighteen hours' worth of stored fuel as glycogen. We all know the other form of stored energy: fat! Presumably, we only store fat if caloric intakes exceed needs, but is that always the case? More later on this juicy tidbit.

In the next phase of its journey, glucose leaves the liver and enters the body's systemic circulation. Here, it becomes available for use by the body's tissues.

A wonderous, complex system of checks and balances manages all of our body's processes. One system in particular regulates how we burn our calories, when we burn them, and when we store them. If the glycogen stored in the liver acts as the coach, calling the plays, the star player is the anabolic hormone *insulin*. Manufactured by your pancreas, insulin controls the metabolism of carbohydrates, lipids, and protein. It directs the pass of available fuel sources for both "team fasting" and "team feeding." When team feeding is up, insulin signals the body to make use of the newly available energy. As insulin is released in response to eating, it has multiple passes to make. One pass is stimulating the storing of energy in the form of glycogen and fat. The other pass is decreasing the amount of glucose made by the liver. The final pass serves to unlock the door and allow entry of glucose into muscle, adipose (fat), and other body tissues.

Factors that can influence the level of glucose in your blood after a meal include:

- how much carbohydrate you consumed
- the digestibility of the carbohydrate consumed
- the amount absorbed by the liver uptake
- the amount of insulin secreted
- how receptive your tissues are to insulin's intended job

Just as insulin signals and calls the shots in the fed state, the other MVP of this game, glucagon, runs plays of its own for the fasted state. Glucagon hits the field when insulin secretion decreases and blood glucose levels drop. Glucagon does the opposite of insulin as it stimulates stored glycogen to be broken back into glucose. By performing in their respective positions properly for team fasting or team feeding, insulin and glucagon are responsible for maintaining the balance of glucose levels in the bloodstream.

The SAD tends to stimulate an overabundance of insulin, helping to drive the problem of insulin resistance in the population. Our goal in sugar detoxing is not necessarily to never stimulate this hormone, but rather to allow your body to release an appropriate amount. Poor-quality foods will trigger a flood of insulin to be released in response to the alarm bells going off as blood sugar levels spike like a five-alarm fire. A balanced, lower-glycemic, higher-fiber, quality meal results in the pancreas responding appropriately and without the stress of averting an emergent situation. A few key points about insulin (especially for those trying to lose weight):

- Insulin secretion inhibits muscle breakdown—a good thing during weight loss.

- Insulin is predominately a storage hormone, which is fine if you need to add some fat tissue, but not so good when you don't need any further deposits into your "fat bank," AKA midsection.

- Insulin blocks fat stores from being accessed for fuel—not so good when you're trying to make a withdrawal from your "fat bank" to use for energy.

- Insulin inhibits fat from being converted into ketones—not so good when you want to burn ketones as a fuel source.

The majority of our body's cells prefer glucose. The brain uses it the most as it's the most easily accessible fuel. Without adequate glucose from food or glycogen stores, the body will turn to backup fuel sources from fats in the form of ketones (a good thing in my opinion) and can even go so far as to catabolize muscle tissue (not a good situation) to convert protein into glucose. The average estimated need for glucose is about 200 grams per day for carb-fueled metabolism. Relax, this book is not a ruse for a hidden keto diet.

The debate on what is better—glucose fueled or ketone fueled— is a topic for another book altogether. But I'll leave this here for you to ponder: one is not necessarily better than the other across the board.

PERSONALIZATION IS KEY

I don't want you to get too wrapped up in macro ratios as we're focusing on weaning off of sugar. I do want you to become more attuned to how your body responds to the improvements in your food choices. Keep a food diary so as you begin to shift toward a lower-sugar diet, you can notice changes in your focus, concentration, sleep, sex drive, energy level, mood, digestion, and bowel habits. Which foods have you feeling satisfied versus sluggish? Are you getting hungry within sixty to ninety minutes of a meal or can you go three to four hours without eating? If you do get hungry too quickly, that's usually a sign that the last meal/snack was insufficiently balanced and most likely was tipped more towards carb, without enough fat or protein to back it up.

When, if at all, are you feeling bloated or gassy? Do feel better with more good fats, moderate protein, and mostly carbs from non-starchy veggies? Or do you feel better when you're predominately plant-powered? Come to the table with an open, beginner's mind and allow your body to tell you precisely what it needs. You may be surprised by its preferences after ignoring the signals for so long or drowning them with sugar.

AN "OVERCALORIED" PEOPLE

While we're on the subject of fuel sources, we should pause for a moment and chat a bit about energy requirements in the form of caloric goals. At present, we are a population of chronically "overcaloried" yet undernourished people. The rates of obesity dictate that we should spend some time discussing it.

According to the CDC and key findings from the National Health and Nutrition Examination Survey released in February 2020:

- In 2017–2018, the obesity rate in adults was 42.4 percent, and there were no significant differences between men and women among all adults or by age group.

- The prevalence of severe obesity in adults was 9.2 percent and was higher in women than in men.

- Among adults, the prevalence of both obesity and severe obesity were highest in non-Hispanic Black adults compared with other races and Hispanic-origin groups.

- The prevalence of severe obesity was highest among adults aged forty to fifty-nine compared with other age groups.

- From 1999–2000 through 2017–2018, the prevalence of both obesity and severe obesity increased among adults.

At this stage of the game, there's no denying that obesity is associated with serious health risks. Morbid obesity only further increases one's risk of obesity-related complications, such as coronary heart disease and end-stage renal disease. Despite all of our knowledge and awareness about the obesity epidemic, the numbers continue to climb. We saw significantly increasing obesity rates from 1999–2000 through 2015–2016.

PREVALANCE OF OBESITY AMONG U.S. ADULTS AGED 20 AND OVER (2017–2018)

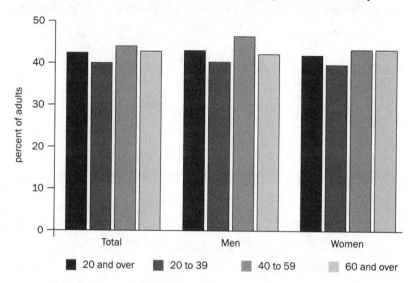

Source: Data from Centers for Disease Control and Prevention, "Prevalence of Obesity and Severe Obesity Among Adults: United States, 2017–2018," updated February 27, 2020, https://www.cdc.gov/nchs/products/databriefs/db360.htm#:~:text=The%20 age%2Dadjusted%20prevalence%20of%20obesity%20was%2042.4%25%2C%20 and,United%20States%20in%202017–2018.

Of note:

• All states and territories had more than 20 percent of adults with obesity.

• Twenty percent to less than 25 percent of adults had obesity in one state (Colorado) and the District of Columbia.

- Twenty-five percent to less than 30 percent of adults had obesity in thirteen states.
- Thirty percent to less than 35 percent of adults had obesity in twenty-three states, Guam, and Puerto Rico.
- Thirty-five percent or more adults had obesity in twelve states.
- The Midwest (33.9 percent) and South (33.3 percent) had the highest prevalence of obesity, followed by the Northeast (29.0 percent) and the West (27.4 percent).
- Six states had an obesity prevalence of 35 percent or higher among non-Hispanic white adults.
- Fifteen states had an obesity prevalence of 35 percent or higher among Hispanic adults.
- Thirty-four states and the District of Columbia had an obesity prevalence of 35 percent or higher among non-Hispanic Black adults.
- Obesity decreased as level of education increased. Adults without a high school degree or equivalent had the highest self-reported obesity (36.2 percent), followed by high school graduates (34.3 percent), adults with some college (32.8 percent), and college graduates (25.0 percent).
- Young adults were half as likely to have obesity as middle-aged adults. Adults aged eighteen to twenty-four years had the lowest self-reported obesity (18.9 percent) compared to adults aged forty-five to fifty-four years, who had the highest prevalence (37.6 percent).

OBESITY IN THE UNITED STATES, 1999–2018

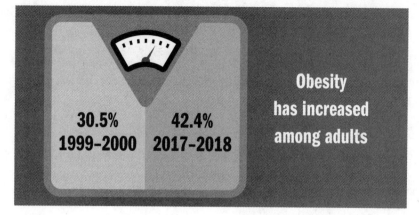

30.5%
1999–2000

42.4%
2017–2018

**Obesity
has increased
among adults**

As this is a book on cutting out the sugar, I have a sneaking suspicion that weight loss or weight maintenance is partly driving your motivation for reading this book. We've all heard, ad nauseum, these two infamous phrases: "If you want to lose weight, you just need to eat less and move more" and "A pound of fat is equal to 3,500 calories, so if you want to lose a pound of fat you need to create a calorie deficit of 3,500 calories." Additionally, and I hate to be the bearer of bad news, but the caloric needs of those of who are fifty and over continue to decrease as age increases. Furthermore, evidence suggests that a degree of caloric restriction is needed to support longevity and anti-aging, so rolling back the calories is not just about weight loss.

DETERMINING YOUR ENERGY REQUIREMENTS

So, what factors should you actually consider when trying to determine your energy requirements? We've long been conditioned to believe that body weight is a clear indication that an individual has been consuming an adequate or inadequate amount of energy. Consume too much energy, you gain weight; consume too little, and weight loss results. That may be true a majority of the time, but in twenty-five years of practice as a functional nutrition clinician, I've seen countless cases where body weight was *not* linked to excessive intakes but was more a result of an imbalanced choice of foods in the diet. Even if you stay within or even slightly below your "appropriate" daily caloric intake, if those calories come from cheap, poor-quality fats and proteins or processed carbs, over time those choices will catch up to you and ultimately be expressed as health issues. Weight gain, digestive issues, brain fog, low libido, joint pain, sleep issues, hormonal imbalance, and impaired detoxification are just some of the issues diet quality influences, regardless of total calories consumed.

While the question of "caloric needs" is not a topic to be skimmed over, I'm not going to belabor the debate regarding the calories-in versus calories-out theory of weight loss (you can read in-depth about this in my other book, *The Stem Cell Activation Diet*). Calories matter to a certain extent, but they are not the end-all-be-all measuring stick for attaining/maintaining a healthy body weight. There's a lot of alphabet soup and abbreviations in the following discussion, but depending on what else you may be reading or what tools/apps you have or will use, it's important to understand the subtle differences. For our purposes here, let's jump to the CliffsNotes on this subject.

The human body burns energy in three forms that add up to your daily total energy expenditure (TEE):

- **Basal energy expenditure (BEE):** how much energy your body needs for basic life processes (this does not include your activities of daily life)

- **Thermic effect of food (TEF):** how much energy your body uses to digest and absorb nutrients from the food you eat
- **Activity thermogenesis (AT):** how much energy your body burns with daily activities and exercise

Basal metabolic rate (BMR), resting metabolic rate (RMR), basal energy expenditure (BEE), and resting energy expenditure (REE) are the four most common terms related to caloric need estimations. BMR and BEE are essentially the same as is RMR and REE. These terms are often used interchangeably, but there are some subtle differences between BMR and RMR. Both BMR and RMR are used to estimate the number of calories you would burn over a twenty-four-hour period at rest. At the end of the day, they all serve a similar purpose, and in nonclinical applications the differences between them will be of little consequence.

The following is a list of factors that can influence your BMR and, in turn, your daily caloric needs:

- **Age.** RMR slows down as we age. So not only does the body require less energy (calories) as we get older, but also you might have to work harder to burn off extras. You may think twice about eating that 100-calorie "snack pack" when you realize it may take you over thirty minutes on the treadmill to burn it off.
- **Body weight.** As your weight decreases, so does your BMR.
- **Environmental temperature.** Yes, it has a small role in BMR, but not as much as you may be hoping for (insert a snarky pun for a rare positive effect of global warming here).
- **Genetics.** They may have a more significant role than you may realize. Consider getting a nutritionally focused genetic panel done to explore this further.

- **Body composition.** Muscle is more metabolically active tissue than fat. Those with more muscle mass will also have higher metabolic rates (something to ponder when determining what type of exercise regimen you want to engage in—cardio vs. strength vs. a combination).

- **How much you exercise.** Get moving—exercise can increase your metabolism.

- **Sex.** Men have an advantage here. BMR is usually higher in men than in women.

- **Health status.** An illness can raise your RMR as your body fights an infection, while nutritional deficiencies can decrease metabolism. (Isn't that a great plug for paying more attention to your nutritional health?)

The following equations are still routinely used to determine caloric needs (and yes, there's an app for them too). Depending on how techy you are, you can either break out the calculator for some old-school math or use one of the many available apps and online tools.

The Original Harris-Benedict Equation

Men BMR = 66.4730 + (13.7516 x weight in kg)
+ (5.0033 x height in cm) – (6.7550 x age in years)

Women BMR = 655.0955 + (9.5634 x weight in kg)
+ (1.8496 x height in cm) – (4.6756 x age in years)

The Revised Harris-Benedict Equation

Men BMR = 88.362 + (13.397 x weight in kg)
+ (4.799 x height in cm) – (5.677 x age in years)

Women BMR = 447.593 + (9.247 x weight in kg)
+ (3.098 x height in cm) – (4.330 x age in years)

The Mifflin–St. Jeor Equation

Men BMR = (10 x weight in kg) + (6.25 x height in cm) – (5 x age in years) + 5 (measured in kcal/day)

Women BMR = (10 x weight in kg) + (6.25 x height in cm) – (5 x age in years) – 161 (measured in kcal/day)

The Harris-Benedict equations have typically been the most commonly used equations to estimate REE. However, these formulas have been criticized for overestimating needs in normal weight and obese individuals by 7 to 27 percent. You may want to either check which equation your app/online tool is using or calculate things the good old-fashioned way using the Mifflin–St. Jeor equation, which studies find to be more accurate.

The majority of foods are rarely made up of one macronutrient, usually bringing a combination of the macros to the party. Our bodies possess the wonderful ability to derive needed fuel from the various macronutrient sources. Like most fuel sources in the world, some are more efficient than others. The same holds true for fuel for the body. Carbohydrates and fats are the most efficient fuels, while protein is not the most effective resource.

PREFERRED CARBOHYDRATES TO FUEL THE BODY

In the process of helping you to lose weight, break the cycle of food addiction, and gain tools for long-term, optimal health, I want to put your mind at ease that we are not here to bash all carbs but to truly appreciate the differences between the sources of carbohydrate. Truth be told, you can survive without carbs. Even the US Food and Nutrition Board's 2005 textbook *Dietary Reference Intakes for Energy, Carbohydrate, Fiber, Fat,*

Fatty Acids, Cholesterol, Protein, and Amino Acids admits that "the lower limit of dietary carbohydrate compatible with life apparently is zero, provided that adequate amounts of protein and fat are consumed."

NON-STARCHY VEGETABLES

Eat the rainbow: dark green, blue, purple, yellow, red, and orange. Local, seasonal, organic, non-GMO is best. Use the EWG resources. Aim for at least six to eight (½ cup cooked, 1 cup raw) servings per day to ensure proper phytonutrient intake to maximize your detox pathways! Choose veggies like:

- artichoke
- arugula
- asparagus
- beets
- bell peppers
- bok choy
- broccoli
- Brussels sprouts
- cabbage
- carrots
- cauliflower
- celery
- collards
- cucumbers
- eggplant
- garlic
- green beans
- kale
- mushrooms
- mustard greens
- okra
- onions
- parsnips
- peas
- peppers (all)
- pumpkin
- radish
- romaine lettuce
- sauerkraut
- seaweed
- spinach
- squashes
- tomatoes
- turnip greens
- watercress

Go easy with starchy vegetables. Try to keep these to one to two times per week.

- acorn squash
- butternut squash
- corn
- plantain
- root vegetables such as beets, carrots, parsnips, potatoes, radishes, rutabaga, sweet potatoes, and yams

LEGUMES

These will also provide fiber and some plant-based protein:

- black beans
- cannellini beans
- edamame
- garbanzo beans/chickpeas
- green lentils
- green peas
- lima beans
- pinto beans
- red lentils

WHOLE GRAINS

If consuming grains, make sure you are choosing whole grains, like the following:

- amaranth
- brown, black, purple, red, or wild rice
- buckwheat
- gluten-free rolled or steel-cut oats
- millet
- nut/seed crackers
- quinoa

FRUITS

Eat whole fruits and try not to drink them. Eat the rainbow. Local, seasonal, organic, non-GMO is best. Use the EWG resources. Aim for one to two servings per day. Consume more vegetables than fruits.

Choose lower-glycemic-index fruits like the following more often:

- all berries
- apples
- lemons
- limes
- oranges
- pears

Choose higher-glycemic-index fruits like the following less often:

- apricots
- bananas
- cantaloupes
- cherries
- coconuts
- figs
- grapefruits
- grapes
- kiwis
- mangoes
- nectarines
- papayas
- peaches
- pineapples
- plums
- pomegranates
- watermelons
- all other fruits

DAIRY AND DAIRY ALTERNATIVES

These can be a source of both carbohydrates and protein.

If consuming dairy, including milk, yogurt, or cheese, opt for organic, grass-fed, and reduced-fat or full-fat, with no artificial sweeteners. During the detox, I recommend choosing dairy alternatives like the following:

- unsweetened cultured yogurt: soy, nut, or coconut
- unsweetened kefir: soy or coconut kefir
- unsweetened plant milks: coconut, almond, cashew, hemp, flax, or hazelnut

PREFERRED FATS TO FUEL THE BODY

Remember, not all fats are bad. Don't be cheap with your fats either—quality rules. For too many years you've been conditioned to believe that all fats are evil. Don't blame the grass-fed butter for what the processed, sugar-laden white bread/bagel/muffin truly did.

- avocados
- oils (extra-virgin, virgin, unrefined, and cold-pressed preferred):

  » almond oil
  » avocado oil
  » butter (grass-fed)
  » coconut oil
  » flaxseed oil

  » ghee
  » macadamia oil
  » olive oil
  » sesame oil
  » walnut oil

- olives
- omega-3 fatty acids from cold-water fish, flax, or chia seeds
- raw, unroasted nuts and seeds and nut butters (these will also provide some protein):

  » almonds
  » Brazil nuts
  » cashews
  » hazelnuts
  » macadamia nuts

  » pecans
  » pumpkin seeds
  » sesame seeds
  » sunflower seeds

PREFERRED PROTEINS TO SUPPORT AND MAINTAIN THE BODY

If consuming animal protein, aim for wild-caught seafood and organic, pasture-raised, hormone-free, antibiotic-free, grass-fed lean meats, poultry, and eggs. Canned fish should be in water and labeled as mercury- and BPA-free. Aim for fish rich in omega-3 fats, such as wild Alaskan salmon, herring, sardines, and black cod. Preferred proteins include the following:

- beef
- bison
- chicken
- duck
- eggs (pastured)
- elk
- fish
- lamb
- turkey
- venison

PLANT-BASED PROTEINS

Choose organic, non-GMO options of the following, if possible:

- dried beans
- dried peas
- lentils
- spirulina
- soy (casein free): tofu, tempeh, edamame, soy milk, soy yogurt

All too often, those with higher body weights are the ones who are the most nutrient deficient. The Standard American Diet (SAD) typically provides an abundance of calorie-dense options without nutrient density—a wasteland devoid of the proper quality fuel with its much-needed micronutrient counterparts that our bodies are literally starving for in order to reach peak performance.

What types of snacks do you reach for when needing a quick pick-me-up? Sugar, caffeine, pretzels, and chips? Besides the usual suspects that we know are just plain unhealthy and full of junk, have you also fallen victim to creative marketing with food masquerading as healthy choices? For example, granola and granola bars, trail mixes, whole grain or even "grain-free" snack chips, and straw- or chip-shaped snacks labeled as "veggies." The majority of these are highly processed and full of sugar. As you review foods to begin limiting and hopefully exclude, reflect on whether these have been frequent fliers in your diet. Are you beginning to see how your body may be desperately craving the changes you are seeking to make?

FOODS TO EXCLUDE OR REDUCE

Proteins: Avoid or reduce your intake of conventionally raised animal proteins, deep-fried protein sources, and processed meat products such as bologna, hot dogs, salami, and sausages.

Carbohydrates: Avoid or reduce your intake of packaged, convenience noodles; processed chips, crackers, and other processed carbohydrates (look for ingredients and fiber content); fried vegetables; and starches. Look out for excess sources of fructose found in table sugar, high-fructose corn syrup, agave syrup, sweeteners, and fruit juices. Limit high-glycemic-index foods. Keep in mind that refined grains behave like simple starches, and since they are easily digested and rapidly absorbed, the rise in blood glucose and subsequent insulin spike can cause the same inflammatory response as sugar.

Fats: Avoid or reduce your intake of processed, damaged trans fats (hydrogenated fats) like those typically found in prepared foods and margarines. Damage can also occur with fat in meats when grilled or broiled on high heat. Avoid fried foods and heat-refined oils.

CHAPTER 4

SUGAR-ADDICTED SOCIETY

Let's argue this case. If we evaluate the facts on how added sugars can contribute to health problems, the following are well-established truths:

- Added sugars are not food.
- Sugars increase the risk of dental caries.
- Excessive intakes of sugars displace needed nutrients and fiber and, therefore, contribute to nutrient deficiencies.
- Sugars contribute to obesity and chronic diseases.
- There is a knowledge deficit in the general public about the types and sources of sugar.
- The average American eats (and drinks) more than 57 pounds of added sugar every year.
- Drinking just one 12-ounce can of soda per day can increase the risk of dying from heart disease by nearly one-third.

- Excess intakes of fructose in added sugar can lead to liver damage similar to that caused by too much alcohol. This is called nonalcoholic fatty liver disease (NAFLD).

- The average American consumes almost three times more added sugar than is recommended per day.

- Sugar is a major cause of chronic inflammation. Inflammation is a root cause of chronic illness and diseases such as diabetes, autoimmune diseases, cardiovascular disease, cancers, arthritis, and neurodegenerative diseases such as Alzheimer's disease.

With stats like that, should sugar be banished instead of fat? The goal here is not to fall from one extreme to the other, as a diet that's too low in carbohydrates will also provide an insufficient amount of nutrients, natural vitamins, and dietary fiber. Remember, we need all of these for optimal health.

Have you ever heard the phrase "What makes you sick also makes you fat, and what makes you fat also makes you sick"? Fat has definitely been the nutrient under fire for decades. As early as the 1950s, the writing on the wall began, pertaining to the impact that sugar was having on the risk of coronary heart disease. Much of that evidence, though, was swept under the proverbial rug for decades, and fat became the scapegoat for the root of all dietary evils.

You may remember hearing in the news back in September 2016 about an article in the September 12, 2016, issue of the *Journal of the American Medical Association*, which exposed the coverup that surrounded the Sugar Research Foundation's (SRF) coronary heart disease research project from 1965. The exposure resulted in a literature review by researchers at the Harvard University School of Public Health Nutrition

Department that was published in 1967 in the *New England Journal of Medicine*. This highly skewed article assigned blame specifically to fat and cholesterol as the causes of coronary heart disease, while purposefully downplaying and casting doubt on the role that sugar intake had as a contributing risk factor. The Harvard-backed study claimed that there was "no doubt" that in order to prevent coronary heart disease, the only change to the American diet that was needed was the reduction of dietary cholesterol and the substitution of polyunsaturated fat for saturated fat. A powerful statement coming from one of the world's most respected universities—setting the stage for the nutrition dogma that has persisted for years.

Contrary to widely accepted practices of ethical standards for research, the SRF's funding and involvement in the project was not disclosed. Over 1,500 pages of documents from the SRF were reviewed and examined that detailed the sugar industry's sponsored research through the 1960s and 1970s that influenced the decision-making of nutrition policy makers, the scientific community, and the general public. To add insult to injury, the sugar industry knew early on that the promotion of a low-fat diet would result in a per-capita increase in consumption of sucrose by at least a third. We all know where the story goes from here: soaring rates of diabetes, heart disease, and obesity. While we will never be able to make up for lost time nor truly quantify the cost impact this misinformation has had, the science is finally catching up and setting the record straight on the role that sugar plays in not only heart disease but also other major chronic diseases.

I wish I could say that this type of industry-sponsored research has only been seen with the sugar industry. However, we see similar issues with the meat, dairy, and egg industries and their armies of lobbyists. All of them sponsor research and then, to varying degrees, selectively cherry-pick data to support their respective platforms. There's a lot of money and politics behind food and nutritional policy making.

Where do we draw the line in the sand regarding a realistic intake of sugar? Currently the American Heart Association (AHA) recommends no more than 9 teaspoons (38 grams) of added sugar per day for men, and 6 teaspoons (25 grams) per day for women. For children, the AHA's recommendations vary depending on age and caloric needs, but between 3 to 6 teaspoons (12 to 25 grams) per day is suggested. The average American consumes anywhere from 17 to 42 teaspoons per day. These numbers can vary depending on influencing factors such as where someone lives, age, gender, and socioeconomic status.

One 20-ounce bottle of the leading cola has a whopping 16 teaspoons of sugar. A beverage that many parents and grandparents give children, apple juice, has 61.8 grams of carbohydrate in a 20-ounce bottle, which is the equivalent of 14.5 teaspoons of sugar. While you may be thinking that 20 ounces of juice is a lot for a child to drink, it the child is not being given water or milk, juices and juice-flavored drinks will be their primary source of hydration. Furthermore, even 10 ounces of apple juice exceeds the recommended amount for children.

Let's look at a drink aimed at consumers of all ages: fruit smoothies. A leading brand of a bottled fruit smoothie has 12 teaspoons of sugar per bottle. Can you see just how easy it is for us to overconsume and fall victim to sugar addictions?

I've mentioned obesity a lot, but that does not mean that those of us at a normal weight are excluded from the impact of sugar. In fact, I often deal with patients whom I would label "skinny fat." They are those who are at a normal body weight or BMI but from a body composition standpoint, their percentage of body fat is disproportionate to their percentage of lean muscle mass, and, if we looked at lab values, they would present with striking similarities to someone who may be labeled overweight or obese and falling into a prediabetic or metabolic syndrome category.

Many people struggling with food addiction are generally dealing with a sugar addiction. Numerous studies have shown the addictive behaviors that high sugar intakes and a diet with high-glycemic foods can trigger. The reason for this is foods with more sugar and their accompanying rapid spike in blood sugar will trigger the area of the brain that is well known for its association with addiction disorders. The technical name of this area is the nucleus accumbens, which we commonly refer to as the pleasure center.

When the pleasure center is triggered, the result is we feel good. Who wouldn't want to continually seek that out? We all like to feel good, right? Yes—but as with all "drugs," the high is usually followed by the crash-and-burn low. Sugar has the power to activate opioid receptors in the brain. We've been hearing so much in the news about opioid addiction regarding medications and drug abuse. If only the same amount of attention were given to the addictive qualities and dependency behaviors that sugar triggers.

I still find it so shocking how little attention has been paid to the fact that sugar has been shown to be *eight times as addictive* as cocaine in rats. Say it aloud with me now: "Sugar has been shown to be eight times more addictive than cocaine!" Time and time again, rat studies on artificial sweeteners, sugar, and even just good ole cookies show the rats choosing these sources of sweetness over addictive drugs like cocaine and morphine. Now, let that sink in. Take a stroll into your kitchen, pantry, or wherever you keep your go-to snack foods. How many of those items are made with refined sugars and processed carbohydrates?

Sadder still, many of us grew up with the food-as-a-reward mentality, a mentality that is still widely practiced today and is a contributing factor to the obesity epidemic that plagues our children. The majority of foods serving as rewards are sugar-based. When is the last time you saw someone dangling a piece of broccoli before a child in an effort to get them to do something? We joke about "dangling carrots" in front of someone to assess their currency for motivation. If only that image were literal. Let's just get it straight right now: food is not a reward; you are not a dog!

SUGAR ADDICTION:
THE PERPETUAL CYCLE

1. Sugar is ingested. It tastes good. You have cravings for it. It triggers addictive responses.

2. Blood sugar rapidly rises. The feel-good hormone dopamine is released in the brain. Your sugar high peaks, and the pancreas releases a flood of insulin to lower blood sugar.

4. Craving and hunger set in with a rapid drop in blood sugar, usually lower than where it started. You crash and burn, which triggers strong cravings and hunger. A vicious cycle repeats.

3. Blood sugar falls quickly. An insulin spike triggers fat storage. The sugar high is fading.

Similar to those who suffer from other addictions, sugar addicts may find themselves facing uncontrollable urges to eat or drink sugary items, even when there is an absence of hunger or in full awareness of wanting to make healthier choices. Foods that spike your blood sugar trigger addiction!

I've been teaching an undergraduate Nutrition for Life course at a local college for a little over five years, and one video that I make my students watch to illustrate the amount of sugar in soda is called "The Happiness Stand." I challenge you to look at it on YouTube (https://youtu.be/X50CFQ9xl-s) and even share it with others.

SUGAR IN BEVERAGES

Sugar is not just in what we are eating but also in what we are drinking. How many calories and grams of sugar do you typically consume each day with your beverage choices? "Diet" beverages don't get a hall pass, either. (We will talk more about sugar substitutes in a bit.)

You may be familiar with the phrase "the latte factor," which is typically a term used for financial planning and budgeting to illustrate monies spent on coffee drinks that could've been invested. But it's also applicable to our discussion on calories and sources of sugar, meaning how are your daily beverage choices fueling your sugar addiction? Even portion sizes have grown significantly over the past few decades. Eight-ounce cans of soda have now been replaced by 12- and 24-ounce bottles. A simple cup of coffee in the 1950s was 6 to 8 ounces. When was the last time you had a 6-ounce serving of any nonalcoholic beverage? Go ahead, I give you permission to insert a snarky comment about drinking plain water here, because in actuality that's probably the most water many Americans are drinking in a day. Sadly, that only further supports the number of excess calories from sugar we are consuming in liquid forms.

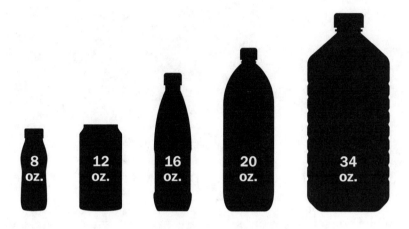

This image shows the evolution of portion sizes over the decades. The problem is that we typically view each of these as a single-serving container. That 16-ounce soda is usually what one person will drink with a meal!

SUGAR PORTIONS IN SODA

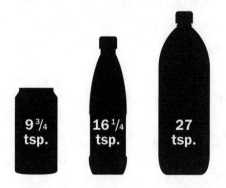

Let's just put things into perspective for those of us who are more visual learners! It's not just sodas here that are concerning. It's all sugar-sweetened beverages, which include sodas, fruit drinks, sports drinks, low-calorie drinks, and any beverage that contains added calories from sweeteners.

TEASPOONS OF SUGAR IN COMMON BEVERAGES

BEVERAGE	SERVING SIZE	TEASPOONS OF SUGAR
Popular colas	20-ounce bottle	17 teaspoons
Orange soda	12-ounce bottle	13 teaspoons
Iced teas	16-ounce carton	13 teaspoons
Popular sports drinks	20-ounce bottle	9 teaspoons
Popular energy drinks	16-ounce can	16 teaspoons

THE YIN AND YANG OF HUNGER HORMONES

Ghrelin and leptin are our hunger and satiety hormones, working as polar opposites in terms of how they affect us. Ghrelin (think growling stomach) stimulates hunger and signals you to begin eating; leptin staves off hunger and tells your brain that you're full and satisfied. Diets high in processed carbohydrates and sugars wreak havoc on the balance of these signaling hormones. This leads to the vicious cycle of hunger and craving with no signs of satisfaction in sight.

Diets rich in sugar, refined and processed carbohydrates, and fructose trigger high levels of insulin to be released and block leptin's ability to signal satiety in your brain. Have you ever experienced feeling hungry shortly after you just consumed an adequate-size or larger meal? If so, that's a prime example of insulin rising and blocking leptin's signaling. Your food choices have now held your body's processes hostage.

To make matters worse, sugars such as fructose are so easily absorbed in the intestinal tract that they bypass some of the checks and balances that glucose would be subjected to and travel directly to the liver. This dose of fructose triggers your liver to convert that sugar directly to fat through a process called lipogenesis, which can lead to nonalcoholic fatty liver disease.

In the presence of a fatty liver, insulin resistance worsens. This is where the system breaks down even further. As your tissue cells become resistant to insulin, the biological response is to increase insulin production, which only sets the stage for it to store more fat.

But insulin and leptin are not the only hormones that are negatively impacted by a diet high in sugar. We already discussed the addictive personality that sugar creates. As with most addictive substances, the addict will develop a level of tolerance over time and will need to consume more of the "drug" in order to get the same effect.

THE SNEAKY SIDE OF SUGAR

One of the major reasons Americans consume so much added sugar is our reliance on packaged convenience in the form of processed foods. Roughly 74 percent of packaged food items contain some amount of added sugars. When you think of added sugars, what's the first thing that comes to your mind? Typical answers would be cakes, cookies, pies, candies, sweets, etc. But what about foods that we don't typically think of as being sweet?

If you look at the ingredient lists of most commercially prepared pasta sauces, you'll find sugar listed as the second or third ingredient. It certainly doesn't help that it's so confusing to read and understand product label claims, ingredient lists, and the nutrition facts label. This issue is part of the reason for the revisions currently being made to the nutrition facts label to help consumers differentiate between sources of naturally occurring sugar and sugars that have been added to a food item. It may be a good exercise for you to take a few minutes poking around your refrigerator and pantries to review the labels of foods that you commonly consume to identify sources of added sugars. A good place to start would be the ketchup bottle, salad dressings, yogurt, and even those granola or fiber bars that you may be using as a "healthy" snack in place of candy.

Did you find any foods that surprised you when you took a deeper look at the ingredients and sugar content? Before beginning any changes to your diet, I encourage you to keep a food journal for a few days of what your typical intake and choices are so that you get an idea of just how much carbohydrate you have been consuming as well as how much of that carbohydrate was coming in the form of added sugars. There are many free online tools and apps to help you with this. Simple and user-friendly options include MyFitnessPal and Carb Manager. Remember, the guidelines are 9 teaspoons (38 grams) of added sugar per day for men and 6 teaspoons (25 grams) per day for women, so do yourself the favor of being honest and transparent with your food diary so you can see exactly how your typical routine measures up against the recommendations.

Sugar is the king of pseudonyms, so it is important to be aware of all of the many different names it can be listed under on an ingredients list. These names include the following:

- agave nectar
- Barbados sugar
- barley malt
- barley malt syrup
- beet sugar
- brown sugar
- buttered syrup
- cane juice

- cane juice crystals
- cane sugar
- caramel
- carob syrup
- castor sugar
- coconut palm sugar
- coconut sugar
- confectioner's sugar
- corn sweetener
- corn syrup
- corn syrup solids
- date sugar
- dehydrated cane juice
- demerara sugar
- dextrin
- dextrose
- evaporated cane juice
- free-flowing brown sugars
- fructose
- fruit juice
- fruit juice concentrate
- glucose
- glucose solids
- golden sugar
- golden syrup
- grape sugar
- HFCS (high-fructose corn syrup)
- honey
- icing sugar
- invert sugar
- malt syrup
- maltodextrin
- maltol
- maltose
- mannose
- maple syrup
- molasses
- muscovado
- palm sugar
- panocha
- powdered sugar
- raw sugar
- refiner's syrup
- rice syrup
- saccharose
- sorghum syrup
- sucrose
- sugar (granulated)
- sweet sorghum
- syrup
- treacle
- turbinado sugar
- yellow sugar

A SPECIAL NOTE ON FRUCTOSE

We've seen a dramatic shift in the amount of fructose being consumed in our diets, as well as the source of it. Previous generations consumed an average of 15 grams of fructose per day, the majority of it in the form of vegetables and fruits. Today, Americans average anywhere from 55 to 75 grams of fructose daily, with the majority of it coming from processed foods and sweetened beverages. Remember, fructose is nearly twice as sweet as glucose. This massive jump in fructose intake is also linked to increases in insulin resistance caused by excess sugar consumption.

High-fructose corn syrup (HFCS) and corn sugar have received a lot of attention over the past few years because they're linked to chronic diseases and obesity. In response, manufacturers have altered the name of corn sugar and sources of fructose on labels. Be on the lookout for names such as:

- natural corn syrup
- isolated fructose
- maize syrup
- glucose/fructose syrup
- tapioca syrup (a non-corn source of fructose)

While our cells can all use glucose for fuel, under normal circumstances, fructose is almost completely metabolized by the liver, which also leads to the production of triglycerides. If your diet is already high in processed, refined, low-fiber carbohydrates, chance are your liver already has ample glycogen stores and excess fructose intake will force it into high-gear fat production. This fat usually ends up finding its way to your midsection.

Another cause for concern is high intakes of fructose have been associated with a decrease in leptin production. Consuming fructose as an added source of sugar will alter your body's ability to signal that you are full.

Does that mean we should throw fruit under the bus because it is also a source of fructose? The differentiating factor here is that fruit is not the empty caloric source of fructose that high-fructose corn syrup is due to the fact that fruit contains fiber and nutrients. The fiber content in whole-food sources of fructose impacts its digestion and absorption.

Another common misconception revolves around fructose's low glycemic response. This is a great benefit when choosing whole food–based sources of fructose but does not justify the use of fructose in the form of added sugars. This is a prime example of how the quality and source of your calories and nutrients matters greatly. You'd be hard-pressed to overeat fructose in the form of whole fruits. Moral of the story here is eat your whole fruits! Exercise caution with drinking fruit juice because you will be missing out on the fiber that the whole fruit would have provided.

WHAT ABOUT THE USE OF ARTIFICIAL SWEETENERS?

If we were trying to eliminate sources of added sugars, it would seem logical that a switch over to artificial sweeteners would be a perfect solution. If only it were that simple. Research has shown that artificial sweeteners can be worse for us than natural sweeteners. Clinical studies have outlined some frightening trends, especially regarding increases in the risk of type 2 diabetes. Areas of concern with use of artificial sweeteners include:

- Artificial sweeteners are far sweeter than regular sugar, which can trigger sugar cravings.

- Because they taste so sweet, you also end up fooling your body into expecting sugar and its source of energy to be en route. In anticipation of this expected dose of sugar, insulin is released. Recall our discussion about insulin also being a fat-storing hormone as part of its job description.

- Artificial sweeteners have been linked with a decreased metabolism and an increased craving for sugar and carbohydrates, especially starchy carbohydrates.

- Artificial sweeteners have been shown to have a negative impact on the gut microbiome.

- Research has demonstrated that those who routinely consume artificial sweeteners also tend to consume more overall calories.

- They're not recommended for use by pregnant and lactating women. That should be justification enough. If there's concern over their safety and use in this population, it stands to reason that we should question their safety for use across all populations.

SUGAR ALCOHOLS

Okay, but what about the pink elephant in the room—the sugar alcohols? Sugar alcohols, which are also known as polyols, are neither sugar nor alcohol. However, their chemical structure resembles a bit of both and they are considered low-digestible carbohydrates (LDCs). Polyols can be found naturally in a variety of fruits and vegetables but are also manufactured from other carbohydrates such as sucrose, glucose, and starch. The most common sugar alcohols found in foods are sorbitol, xylitol, mannitol, maltitol, maltitol syrup, lactitol, erythritol, isomalt, and hydrogenated starch hydrolysates. While most sugar alcohols are approximately half as sweet as sucrose, maltitol and xylitol are equally as sweet as sucrose.

The sugar alcohols can contribute to gas, bloating, and even diarrhea in some individuals due to their slow and incomplete absorption in the intestinal tract. (If you're ever in need of a good laugh, look up the Amazon reviews for Haribo sugar-free gummy bears.) It's this incomplete absorption that makes them attractive as a sweetener, as they have little effect on your blood sugar when compared to glucose, and insulin is not stimulated by their consumption. Erythritol, notably, has been shown to be better tolerated than the others in this class. The caloric contribution of the sugar alcohols can range from 0 to 3 calories per gram (kcal/g). While the sugar alcohols are in a class all their own under the umbrella of alternatives to sugars, the issue that remains persistent with their use is the overall triggering of cravings for sweetness. When our goal is to help you break the cycle of sugar cravings, it's best to eliminate all the roadblocks, and that includes artificial sweeteners, non-nutritive sweeteners, sugar alcohols—the entire lot!

CHAPTER 5

WHY DO I NEED TO DETOX?

Does your personal motivation to detox include prevention or improvement of health problems such as diabetes, obesity, higher blood pressure, and inflammation? Maybe you're more focused on healthy aging and prevention of cognitive disorders like Alzheimer's disease, which is now being increasingly referred to as type 3 diabetes, as insulin resistance in the brain is strongly linked to cognitive dysfunction.

Whatever your motivation, merely uttering the word "detox" could have you cringing and standing at the ready to debate the separation of science and pseudoscience. I completely understand the reason for this, as "detox" is a term that usually has me ready for battle. The world of "Doctor Google" combined with the never-ending stream of unqualified quacks has completely adulterated the term and undermines the efforts of those of us who subscribe to evidence-based, science-backed, functional medicine practices. What makes this book different is that we will be using the proven science behind nutrient-dense food to provide the tools for detoxing rather than some marketing gimmick in a flowery package. Food is powerful medicine!

Detoxes have been gaining in popularity in recent years, and it seems as if each week a new detox tea, potion, or concoction hits the shelves or your inbox and social media streams. Then there are the 2 a.m. infomercials selling detox or cleanse programs promising to deliver the fountain of youth or a bounty of related benefits. Truth is, the majority of these programs and products are not necessary to perform a detox or cleanse. You can't simply detox poor diet and lifestyle choices.

"DETOX" DEFINED

Simply put, detoxification, also known as biotransformation, is the body's natural process of breaking down and removing substances that are unwanted and present the potential to cause harm. These can be waste products produced by the body or externally sourced items such as medications, environmental toxins, or any substances that can be ingested, inhaled, or absorbed. The process of detoxification is handled continuously (and in most cases effectively) by the major organs of detoxification: the liver, GI tract, kidneys, lungs, and the largest organ of the body, the skin. The circulatory and lymphatic systems also assist with transport and removal of waste products.

Detoxification is not just a physiological process but a psychological one too, as habits and patterns can also benefit from a review of one's social, emotional, and spiritual well-being. For example, with the reliance on social media and electronics, you may hear the phrase "device detox." The psychological side of detox is so important to maintaining balance in these systems. When it comes to "sugar detox," the psychological side is just as important to long-term success as the physiological side.

Detoxification is a very complex process heavily reliant on nutrients, as illustrated below. You can see exactly how many different compounds are necessary in order to appropriately detoxify the body.

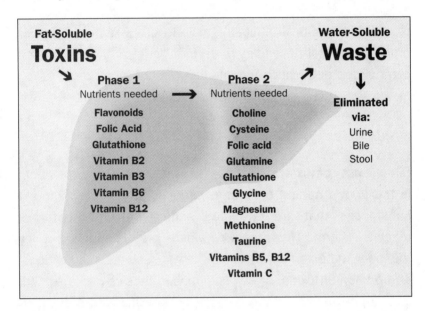

BIOTRANSFORMATION EXPLAINED

THE LIVER

Your liver plays the starring role in the detox process, filtering the blood that passes through and removing chemicals, dead cells, drugs, microorganisms, and other waste debris. The removal of debris is an intricate process requiring micronutrients, such as B vitamins, to fuel the reactions to take place. Effective detoxification also requires amino acids and other vitamins.

Poor diet, with intakes high in sugars and damaged, poor-quality fats, have impaired liver function for many. The rates of people diagnosed with "fatty liver," nonalcoholic steatohepatitis, and nonalcoholic fatty liver should help to illustrate the masses of those suffering with impaired detox abilities. It's worth noting that the latter is the more severe of the two and is associated with inflammation, obesity, and metabolic syndrome.

If left untreated, fatty liver disease can lead to cirrhosis as scarring builds up in the liver tissue. Be sure to show your liver a little love and help support it to thrive and heal. The liver is a miraculous organ capable of regeneration and possesses the ability to respond positively to diet and lifestyle changes. If you've been struggling with liver concerns, hope is not lost. The sooner changes are made the faster the road to liver recovery.

The primary goals for addressing a fatty liver are lifestyle and diet changes. Refrain from alcohol, lose weight, and improve blood sugar control. High-fructose corn syrup is no friend to the liver and should be completely eliminated.

THE KIDNEYS

The kidneys are also a costar in the detox production. They also remove waste products and toxins from the blood and follow up with excretion into the urine. The skin and lungs play supporting roles in biotransformation. The lungs filter and remove other waste products, and our skin eliminates waste products and toxins in our sweat. Maybe you know someone who thought sweating it out in a sauna was just to help with weight loss. Well, indirectly, it can, as saunas support the detoxification process by promoting sweating. Many people struggling with weight issues may also be dealing with inefficiencies in their detox pathways. Remember our discussion on being overcaloried and undernourished? Nutrients are necessary for effective biotransformation; if you're nutrient deficient, the effectiveness of detoxification will be reduced.

Why, then, is there so much debate surrounding detoxification? Yes, we do have all of the tools necessary within our bodies to perform detoxification. However, possession of a tool does not always equate to its effectiveness to complete a task. Such is the case with detoxification for so many, as we continue to subject our bodies to an ever-increasing polluted and stressful environment, which can impose extra burdens upon this system, straining its efficiency.

Stressors impacting the body's detoxification capabilities include:

1. At the top of the list is diet and excessive exposure to and consumption of high-fructose corn syrup, trans fats, caffeine, alcohol, and processed, refined foods. These are considered "antinutrients."

2. Medications, including having them too much, too often, or with inappropriate or improper use.

3. Toxins formed as part of the metabolic process, such as nitrogen, carbon dioxide, bile, urea, free radicals, and stool.

4. External exposure to the following toxins:

- heavy metals such as mercury, arsenic, lead, cadmium, tin, and aluminum

- indoor pollutants such as flame retardants and mycotoxins from mold exposure

- chemicals including pesticides, herbicides, cleaning products, solvents, glues, cosmetics, and toiletries

- allergens in food, mold, dust, pollen, and chemicals
- potentially infectious organisms such as bacteria, viruses, yeast, and parasites
- xenobiotics in preserved meats, charred/high-temperature-cooked foods, food additives, sugar, and pesticides
- outdoor pollutants
- chlorinated/fluoridated drinking water

Take a moment here to pause and review these four barriers to detoxification. Ask yourself how much of a role they may be playing in your life.

The following psychological factors can also influence the presence of toxins in the body:

1. No surprise here to see stress topping the list. How often do you feel stressed by too much work, not enough play time, lack of quality sleep, worrying about finances, family, etc.?

2. Issues impacting mental health, such as addictions, overeating, and detrimental mental patterns like negative self-talk.

3. Media input overload. Are you being overstimulated by devices?

4. Connectedness. Do you lack a spiritual connection or feel a lack of meaning and purpose in your life? Do you ever struggle with feelings of isolation? Do you have adequate social support and a sense of community and belonging?

5. Nature deprivation. How often are you deprived the opportunity to connect with your natural environment?

6. Negativity. Do you often find yourself experiencing negative emotions and engaging in negative self-talk, or experiencing feelings such anger, fear, guilt, and hopelessness?

SIGNS OF A STRUGGLING DETOX SYSTEM

How can you tell if your body's detoxification pathway is hitting some bumps in the road? Are your biotransformation processes just limping along? Take a look at the following list of potential signs and symptoms. If there is no other medical explanation for their presence in your life, it may be time to take a deeper look at the efficacy of your body's ability to clean house.

- adrenal fatigue
- bad breath
- brain fog
- dark circles under the eyes
- fatigue
- fluid retention
- foul body odor
- foul-smelling stools and dark-colored urine
- frequent colds and persistent infections
- gas, bloating, and IBS-type issues
- headaches
- heartburn
- hormonal issues
- infertility
- joint pain
- loss of muscle tone
- low libido
- mood changes
- muscle aches
- premature aging
- sinus congestion and postnasal drip
- skin issues like rashes and canker sores
- sleep issues
- weight changes, excess weight

If any of these lists have rung a few bells for you, the next question you may be asking yourself is "What do I need do to feel better?"

IMPROVING DETOX PATHWAYS

Now you know just how important the digestive system is to detoxification. From a functional medicine perspective, the GI system is the control center for the rest of the body and is responsible for far more than simply digesting, absorbing, and eliminating the foods we eat. The surface area of your intestinal lining is approximately 4,305 square feet and requires about 40 percent of your body's energy expenditure. Poor GI health sets a downward spiral in motion, leading to the body's inability to maintain homeostasis, or balance, and to the decline of other bodily systems. In my opinion, there is not a single health condition or disease that does not link back to the functional health of the gut.

Your gut flora, which make up your individual microbiome, reside within this wondrous GI system. The GI tract is home to roughly 70 percent of your body's immune system, providing you with a protective barrier against microorganisms and antigens. Antigens influence the body's reactions to foods and, therefore, play an important role in the development of food sensitivities, inflammatory conditions, chronic diseases, and yes, the efficacy of detoxication. The GI tract is also the production source for approximately two-thirds of your body's hormones and neurotransmitters. Take a moment to consider how you would rate the overall health of your digestive system, as this can also provide you with some insight to possible roadblocks to biotransformation.

WHAT'S IN MY GENES?

I just want to take a moment here to briefly discuss the genetic relationship to detoxification. I mentioned earlier that opponents of detoxification programs will claim that our bodies do not need any help with detoxification because we are already well equipped with the organs of detoxification, and our cells possess all the tools they need to complete this process day in and day out. This theory would be correct—if the individual is healthy. But as we have discussed at length, the current population suffers a high degree of unhealthfulness.

As the knowledge and understanding of the human genome has grown, the science of nutrigenetics, or the study of how a person's genes impact their need for and utilization of a specific nutrient, illustrates how people who appear overall as "healthy" may have variations in their genes that can greatly impact their detoxification processes. Researchers are exploring how some gene variants can correlate with disease, drug response, and other phenotypes.

This means that the function of the enzymes of the detoxification pathways may be compromised in individuals as result of certain gene variants. Through the power of food, nutrigenomic interventions can provide support by upregulating the expression of those genes to aid the detoxification process and, ultimately, benefit the person with the variants. We could devote an entire book just covering this topic; if you're interested in learning more, I encourage you to explore the free content on the Genetic Science Learning Center website provided by the University of Utah. You can access it at https://learn.genetics.utah.edu/content/basics. Direct-to-consumer genetic tests are widely available and less cost-prohibitive than they were just a few years ago. I would encourage you to work with a reputable evidence-based company, preferably one that requires a licensed, trained clinician to order and interpret the test results for you.

BENEFITS OF A SUGAR DETOX

If you're still wavering a bit about taking this change on, let's just review some of the benefits awaiting you on the other side of breaking free from sugar's grasp.

Improved metabolism and overall body function. You'll be consuming foods that are nutrient dense, not calorically dense. It's time to get nourished! You'll be bidding goodbye to sugary foods that are devoid of vitamins and minerals.

Increased energy, with fewer overall calories. Nutrient-dense vegetables and fruits combined with protein and healthy fats will keep you not only energized without the "crashing" feeling, but also feeling fuller longer without having to feel deprived.

Increased cognitive function. No more brain fog! Your brain will now be getting its fuel from healthy sources, which aids with its peak performance.

Clearer, younger-looking skin. Just because this book is aimed at the 50+ crowd does not mean that you aren't struggling with acne. Acne can be caused by a hormonal imbalance that is driven by sugar consumption. Less sugar = less acne. Excess sugar in your diet causes glycation, a process where free radicals can attack the proteins collagen and elastin in your skin, leading to premature aging and wrinkles. Less sugar = healthier overall skin.

Weight loss. Time to shed those extra pounds, and if they've been hanging around your midsection, then sugars have given you an outward sign of how they work against you. Some of it will also be water weight, so you may notice that you're not as puffy or retaining as much fluid.

Improved hormonal balance. Hormones regulate your metabolism. Sugar has negative effects on your hormones, such as insulin, leptin, ghrelin, and sex hormones.

Reduced inflammation and disease risk. Inflammation is a root cause of illness, and sugar triggers a cascade of proinflammatory chemicals. Cutting out the sugar will lead to an anti-inflammatory effect, which not only benefits healthy aging, brain function, and chronic pain, but also reduces your risk of chronic diseases, especially diabetes, cardiovascular disease, and fatty liver.

Improved glycemic control. Whether or not you have already been diagnosed with type 2 diabetes, pre-diabetes, metabolic syndrome, or insulin resistance, cutting out the sugar will take the stress off of the pancreas and regulatory hormones trying to handle all of that sugar. Those on medications to control blood sugar may have to work with a prescriber on dosage adjustments as blood sugar levels improve and even normalize with the diet and lifestyle change associated with this program.

Healthier microbiome. You can improve the cultural population and diversity of microbes in your gut in as little as three days! A healthy gut = a happy gut = balance. Relapsing back to your old diet will result in the microbial changes reverting back = imbalance.

CHAPTER 6

HOW DO I BEGIN LETTING GO OF SUGAR?

Are you ready to take the first step toward breaking the cycle of addiction to sugar? I mentioned in the beginning of the book that there would be one quiz. Well, get ready, it's quiz time! Set some time aside, grab a pen, and commit to being totally honest with yourself as you go through the following twenty questions. Topic: SUGAR!

20 QUESTIONS ABOUT MY USE OF SUGARS

Simply answer **yes** or **no** to each of the following questions. Be honest!

	Yes	No
1. I eat refined sugars and processed carbohydrates every day.	☐	☐
2. I have been teased about being "addicted" to sugar or carbs.	☐	☐
3. Thoughts of cutting out sugar or carbs make me nervous, anxious, or stressed.	☐	☐
4. I cannot go a day without eating or drinking something sweet.	☐	☐
5. I have hidden sugar-containing items to consume in private.	☐	☐
6. I feel tired or achy after I consume refined sugars and processed carbohydrates.	☐	☐
7. I eat even when I am not hungry.	☐	☐
8. I get hangry if I don't eat every few hours.	☐	☐
9. There are certain foods that I cannot control myself around.	☐	☐
10. I feel guilty at times about what I have eaten.	☐	☐
11. When I am stressed, I immediately reach for sugar.	☐	☐
12. I have tried cutting out sugar more than once in the last twelve months.	☐	☐
13. I use food as a reward.	☐	☐

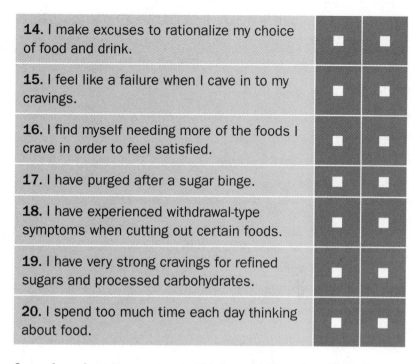

	Yes	No
14. I make excuses to rationalize my choice of food and drink.	◼	◼
15. I feel like a failure when I cave in to my cravings.	◼	◼
16. I find myself needing more of the foods I crave in order to feel satisfied.	◼	◼
17. I have purged after a sugar binge.	◼	◼
18. I have experienced withdrawal-type symptoms when cutting out certain foods.	◼	◼
19. I have very strong cravings for refined sugars and processed carbohydrates.	◼	◼
20. I spend too much time each day thinking about food.	◼	◼

One of my favorite quotes is "Not everything that is faced can be changed. But nothing can be changed until it is faced," by James Baldwin. Take a moment to let that sink in as you reflect on your answers to the quiz.

How did you do? If you answered yes to four or more questions, it is definitely a worthwhile endeavor to assess your relationship with sugar and refined processed carbohydrates. I know it may seem daunting and scary, but believe me, your future self is going to thank you for the steps that you're going to be taking toward returning balance to your body. Right here and now, let me be the first to congratulate you on taking this very important step forward.

Keep that pen and pad handy because we're going to need it a bit longer. While we only had the one quiz to take, there are a few exercises I'd encourage you to complete as part of the prep work for sugar detox. We covered that detoxing encompasses both the physiological and the psychological domains. These exercises will help prep you for the psychological side of the detox.

Making changes always requires a degree of determination, preparation, planning, and ultimately, commitment to the change. When embarking upon a change that requires quitting a substance that you crave or even feel addicted to, the commitment becomes even more important. As mentioned in Chapter 2, the definition of insanity is "doing the same thing over and over and expecting a different response." Now I am asking you to ponder this definition and how many times you have tried different versions of essentially the same thing. Ask yourself these questions now:

What has worked for you in the past, and what has not worked for you with previous attempts at making dietary or lifestyle changes?

What was it about the previous changes you were trying to make that made them unsustainable for the long haul?

I'd like you to jot down the answers here:

Take a moment to assess your readiness for change. This is a significant undertaking that you're embarking upon. I'm not going to begin spewing some twelve-step program philosophy or have you recite the serenity prayer (although I really happen to like the message there), but instead will offer tools and resources to assist you to be a successful changemaker.

READY FOR A CHANGE?

I've been working with clients one-on-one for over twenty-five years, and two of the most powerful tools in my arsenal are helping them identify their readiness for change and mapping out a goal-planning strategy. One reason why people fail often with diets is they jump headfirst into the shallow end of the change pool rather than landing on their feet. Sometimes, in the excitement of choosing to finally make a change, we get a bit overzealous and a bit ahead of ourselves, which generally leads to a quick start and an even quicker quitting of a program. That's another reason why the game plan for weaning you off of sugar is in fact a *weaning* program rather than an abrupt stop, despite the insinuations of the term "detox."

Now, I'd like you to read through the following descriptions of the different stages of change and ask yourself which stage you would place yourself in.

Stage 1: Pre-contemplation. When in this stage, individuals probably aren't even considering making lifestyle changes. Or, it may be on the radar, but they can't picture themselves doing it anytime soon. You are reading this book, so chances are you're already past this stage.

Stage 2: Contemplation. In this stage, individuals are seriously considering changing their lifestyle but aren't totally committed. They might be weighing the pros and cons of changing but struggling with the amount of time and energy required for success.

Stage 3: Preparation. They're getting closer and more serious about making some changes and have made a commitment to try to change in the next thirty days. They might also have attempted to change at least one other time in the past year but were still not where they would like to be.

Stage 4: Action. Alright, they're in the thick of it now. They are actively making lifestyle changes, have experienced some success, and are committed to a healthier lifestyle.

Stage 5: Maintenance. Hooray! For the most part, they have been engaged in a healthy lifestyle for the past six months or more, and new, sustained behaviors have emerged. They have every intention of continuing for the long haul.

There is a Stage 6: Relapse. The individual returns to old behaviors and abandons the new changes. If this occurs, it's time to evaluate the triggers for relapse and reassess the motivation and barriers to change.

I am currently in Stage:

In order to move up to the next stage, I would need:

A few more points of consideration to assist you with determining your level of readiness:

Are you motivated to change your lifestyle to improve your health?

....

And if so, how motivated are you on a scale of 1 to 5?

....

Are you planning to make the changes in the next thirty days?

....

Do you agree that small, gradual changes are the best approach to long-term success?

....

Is there anything in your life right now or over the next six months that could act as a barrier to your success?

....

....

Do you have a support system of family or friends who will be in favor of your effort to change? If so, who?

....

....

Are you willing to commit the effort required to achieve your diet and lifestyle goals?

....

Now that you've invested some time focusing on your readiness for change, it's time to begin creating your strategy for success through vision planning and goal setting.

Take some time here to answer the following questions:

Where do you want to be in three to five years regarding your health, well-being, and quality of life? Describe the big picture you have in mind for yourself.

....

....

....

....

I want you to imagine feeling the way you want to feel and looking the way you want to look. Describe the possibilities here.

....

....

....

....

How do you see your life being different as a result of the changes to your diet and lifestyle when you achieve your health goals?

....

....

....

....

What may need to be different in your life right now for you to make your health a priority?

....

....

....

....

Describe what a healthy lifestyle means to you.

....

....

....

....

What is one thing that you can do today to begin living a healthier lifestyle?

....

....

....

....

List the changes you intend to make that you will be able to sustain over time.

....

....

....

....

PLAN AND PREP: DIFFERENT KINDS OF FOUR-LETTER WORDS

Failure to plan is planning to fail, so the more time you can devote to planning and preparing for the changes you want to make, the more likely you are to be successful. Another key factor in the planning component is setting a target date, so take the time to look at your work and social schedules, and discuss things with your family or friends. Choose a start date when you know there will be few or no events that may present temptations too early on in your detox plan.

The next step is goal planning. The key to setting goals is to personalize them according to the uniqueness of your own circumstances and individual needs. The purpose of goal setting is to map out a specific plan for achieving them. I have routinely encouraged my clients to use the SMART method for establishing goals, and I suggest the same for our purposes here as well. Remember, a goal without a plan is just a wish! Once you create a goal, it's important to take a pulse on it routinely so you can track your progress. Also, while you may have a broader goal, consider narrowing it down into more bite-sized, measurable chunks, like stepping stones bridging where you are to where you want to be.

SMART goals are:

- Specific
- Measurable
- Action-oriented and Adaptable
- Realistic
- Tangible

Try to limit the actual number of goals to no more than three, but one or two are just fine. Now, give it a try by listing your goals and plans for achievement. You may want to consider goals pertaining to diet, exercise, lifestyle factors, and self-care, or even exploring a new interest or hobby as part of your detox process. The sky's the limit. The wonderful thing about these exercises is that you can apply them to any aspect of your life.

If you're not quite ready yet to create your goal statements, that's fine too. You might want to finish reading through the entire book first. If that's the case, feel free to come back to these pages at a later time. Just do yourself the favor of working through the exercise.

Be sure to make your goals specific and use positive, affirming language, such as "I can," "I will," and "I am." Create your plan with determination but also realism and flexibility. Then, compare your statement against the SMART acronym to help cement them.

Goal 1:

....

Plan for achievement:

....

....

....

Goal 2:

....

Plan for achievement:

....

....

....

Goal 3:

....

Plan for achievement:

....

....

....

PREPARING FOR THE POTENTIAL OF SUGAR WITHDRAWAL

I don't want to do you the injustice of sugarcoating things here. There's a strong possibility that you will experience withdrawal symptoms. The extent and degree of symptoms that you may experience can vary depending on how long you've been consuming excessive amounts of sugar and how much you typically consumed per day. We have discussed the science behind the addictive qualities of sugar at length, so in preparation for that, you need to acknowledge that you may be embarking on one of the most difficult breakups that you have faced in your life. Many times, the barrier between addiction and freedom from addiction can't be broached due to fear of the detox process. In regard to sugar, the withdrawal symptoms and detox process can be somewhat uncomfortable, but with proper planning, support, and help, your sugar detox does not need to be an insurmountable task.

SYMPTOMS OF WITHDRAWAL

As I mentioned above, symptoms can vary from person to person, ranging from mild to very strong. Withdrawal symptoms will usually present themselves within one to two days after your last meal or snack that contained sugar. Symptoms may persist for a few days or may last up to a week. As our plan is more of a weaning than an abrupt stopping of all carbs, you are likely to experience less drastic symptoms than what could be expected with more rigorous programs.

Breaking up with sugar will take more than sheer willpower due to the physiological effect sugar has on the body and the brain. Sugar triggers the brain's production of dopamine, one of the feel-good reward-center chemicals, which is why we want and crave sugary foods and drinks.

Possible psychological withdrawal symptoms include:

- changes in mood, such as anxiety, depression, becoming easily agitated, or restlessness
- changes in sleep patterns
- hunger and intense cravings for sugar
- difficulty with focus and concentration

Possible physiological withdrawal symptoms include:

- headaches
- fatigue
- feeling faint or dizzy
- joint or muscle aches or pains
- weight changes
- chills and flu-like symptoms

- gas and bloating
- changes in bowel habits
- nausea

Tips for reducing withdrawal symptoms:

- Don't quit cold turkey. Gradually step down your sugar intake.
- Drink plenty of water.
- Use exercise and movement to promote endorphin release to keep you feeling good and energized.
- Allow for time to get some extra sleep.
- For cravings, add flavors to your foods and snacks through herbs, spices, or even bitters, as these can help to direct your tastes away from sweet-seeking.

Keep in mind that being forewarned is to be forearmed, so begin to prepare for the possibility of experiencing these symptoms and formulating a plan for how you will manage them.

CHAPTER 7

ARMED AND READY: PUTTING TOGETHER MY OWN DETOX PLAN

As you aim to take over the reins to your health, pause for a moment to review any risk factors that may increase your chance of getting a disease. Risk factors fall into two categories: modifiable or unmodifiable. Examples of unmodifiable risk factors include age, gender, ethnic background, and family history. When it comes to modifiable risk factors, our lifestyle choices are key influences on our overall health, wellness, and susceptibility to disease. Modifiable risk factors include smoking, high blood pressure, insulin resistance, pre-diabetes, diabetes, physical inactivity, being overweight, and high blood cholesterol.

DIETARY SUPPORT OF BIOTRANSFORMATION

Of course, making better food choices, as follows, will be at the top of any list of ways to better support sugar detoxification:

The DOs

- Consume whole foods.

- Prepare most of your meals at home.

- Stay hydrated. Drink at least six to eight glasses of filtered water a day. Water is not only the fluid of life, it is also vital for removal of toxins.

- Make fiber one of your new best friends. Aim for 25 to 30 grams per day. We're aiming for one to two bowel movements a day—not every other day, and certainly not per week. Moving your bowels is the body's way of taking out the trash; thus, if you're not moving your bowels regularly, waste and toxins are hanging out in the intestinal tract, making you even more toxic.

- Eat a more plant-forward diet consisting of organic, non-GMO produce as much as possible. Choose legumes (preferably cooked to reduce and eliminate lectins, which can be problematic for some). Choose whole grains (preferably gluten-free). Include plenty of non-starch vegetables, fruits, nuts, and seeds.

- Include fermented foods to provide natural sources of probiotics.

The DON'Ts

- Do not consume the foods that can damage the gut: gluten, dairy, and sugar.

» Gluten consumption can damage the production of a protein called zonulin, which is a necessary component in maintaining the integrity of the junctions between cells in the lining of the intestines.

» Dairy can be proinflammatory for many people, so it is a good idea to avoid it when trying to repair and prevent damage to your gut.

» Excess sugar in the diet feeds the bad bacteria in the gut, causing an imbalance of flora and bacterial overgrowth known as dysbiosis. This greatly contributes to the erosion of gut permeability.

- Do not subject food to high-temperature cooking, such as frying and deep frying.
- Do not cook with PTFE-coated nonstick pans.
- Do not drink water or drinks from plastic bottles unless they are guaranteed to be BPA-free. Use glass bottles or even a Mason jar.
- Do not store food in plastic containers or cover food in plastic wrapping. Use glass or earthenware instead. Never reheat food in plastic!
- Do not microwave your food.
- Do not consume processed foods.

LIFESTYLE SUPPORT OF BIOTRANSFORMATION

- Avoid exposure to the known toxicants we discussed earlier. This includes evaluating your choices of personal care and household cleaning products.

- Breathe clean air. Consider the use of HEPA or ULPA filters.

- Break a sweat regularly. Get moving with exercise, use steam baths, and use saunas.

- Get and stay moving on a regular basis. This includes physical activity and exercise, yoga, tai chi, dancing, and anything you enjoy that gets you moving and increases your heart rate.

- Schedule time for manual therapies. Go for a massage; try acupuncture. Massage can improve lymph flow and help the body with elimination of toxins.

- Spend time in nature, and get grounded. Yes, that means allowing your bare feet to walk in the grass for a bit.

- Get connected, and not in the electronic way. Unplug and spend time with family and friends, and engage in activities that foster a sense of community.

- Explore other self-care practices that may resonate with you, such as meditation, journaling, breathing techniques, guided imagery, and visualization.

READY TO ROLL! YOUR DETOX ACTION PLAN

Here we go. You've planned and prepped, chosen your food-logging tool, maybe even used the calculators we covered to determine some macronutrient goals. Now it's time to implement. Here's the play-by-play outline for successfully detoxing from sugar and building long-lasting change.

STEP 1: TAKE INVENTORY. WHAT'S IN YOUR KITCHEN?

"Out of sight, out of mind" may be your mantra to refrain from sugar, but if it's still in the house, you may be tempted to seek it out. Now, I'm not suggesting that you completely tear your home apart, throwing away bags of food, but you may want to give yourself a leg up on success and do a little sugar spring cleaning before starting. Consider removing all processed, refined, and junk foods to make room for healthy, nourishing foods that you will be choosing in place of sugar.

A toast—let's drink to your health and new lease on a life in balance.

STEP 2: ADEQUATE HYDRATION. DRINK CLEAN, FILTERED WATER

Aim for: half of your body weight in ounces. If you are currently obese, then opt for using an adjusted body weight. Drink water throughout the day, not just with meals. Caffeine-containing beverages, such as coffee, soda, and tea, have a diuretic effect, resulting in the body losing more water than is ingested, so they should not be your primary source of fluid intake.

Avoid alcohol. Not only does it act as a bit of a diuretic, but it also inhibits your organs of detoxification—not what you want during a detox plan. Fruit juices are too high in sugar; therefore, they are not a recommend choice for detoxification. Okay, I'm sure you're thinking, "Well, what about smoothies?" Avoid the commercially prepared ones, and if making your own, make sure the smoothie is predominantly vegetables and a small bit of fruit. I do not recommend using a juicer that extracts the juice and separates out the fiber. Instead, opt for a high-powered blender that will retain the fiber. Fiber is your new best friend and extremely important in obtaining optimal gastrointestinal health and decreasing the rate of absorption of sugars.

STEP 3: FOOD CHOICES. FOCUS ON QUALITY FIRST, THEN QUANTITY

Start the day off on the right foot. If you are choosing to consume breakfast, be sure your breakfast provides a balance of our three macronutrient groups: carbohydrates, proteins, and fats. A common mistake is starting the day off with an extremely high load of carbohydrates in the form of breakfast cereals, breakfast bars, smoothies, and the gamut of breakfast bakery items that are loaded with sugar and made with refined flours. Plus, top it all off with a supersized cup of coffee with a processed creamer and sweetener, and you'll be first in line for the insulin roller coaster. A choice like that would set you up for a sugar craving within a couple of hours.

As you go through your day, pay attention to the signals your body is sending you. How are you feeling? What's your level of focus and concentration? Are you hungry or thirsty? When you first begin scaling back sources of sugar, focus on the timing of and between your meals and snacks. Try not to let yourself go longer than four hours, as that can set the craving coaster in motion. It's always a good idea to make sure that you have some healthy snack options with you at all times in case of schedule changes or any of life's other curveballs. Don't forget the recipe resources at the end of the book! You will always have a healthy option on hand to carry you through to your next meal. This will help prevent you from choosing a food that is not in alignment with your goal or pushing your hunger scale to the brink and putting you in a position where you may fall victim to a poor choice. Nuts and seeds are a great option to consider here because they travel well all year long, regardless of the climate.

Later in the day, try to make dinner a light meal, not the typical heavy one that has you feeling bloated and heavy the rest of the night. There are loads of great dinner recipes for you to try out at the end of the book. Get in the habit of not eating anything for two to three hours before bed. Take it one step further by layering in a mild fast, keeping twelve hours between your last intake at night and the first intake of the next day.

STEP 4: A BODY IN MOTION STAYS IN MOTION

We literally could devote an entire chapter to the benefits of movement and physical activity. Movement can serve multiple purposes in support of our detoxing goal. To detox through the skin, choose activities that cause you to break a sweat. Movement and exercise also release feel-good hormones, and during sugar withdrawal, you will want a source of these endorphins to replace the sugar high. Exercise is also a great way for your body to burn glycogen, and to tap into your sugar reserves that have been converted into and stored as fat. If you have not worked out for some time, start slow and gradually increase the amount of activity each day. Begin with one to two 10-minute chunks per day that raise your heart rate and gradually increase the frequency, duration, and intensity of your movement activities.

Additionally, exercise is great for relieving stress and helping you to sleep better. When sleep and stress are out of balance, biochemical pathways unfortunately stimulate cravings for carbohydrates and sugars. That's the perfect segue to our next two steps.

STEP 5: ADDRESS YOUR STRESS

If your typical response to stress has been to self-medicate with food, be sure to explore other options prior to beginning the sugar detox. The body triggers mobilization of glucose as part of the fight-or-flight response. For many of us in today's society, dealing with chronic stress causes this system to go on the fritz and can be an underlying driver of chronic sugar cravings. Consider other stress-relieving tools, such as deep breathing, reading, listening to music, spending time with family or friends, or caring for an animal; or other integrative approaches, such as meditation, acupressure, guided imagery, and tapping (also known as Emotional Freedom Technique). Just as you will want to have a snack on hand with you at all times, it is also a good idea to consider what your emergency stress stopper(s) will be.

STEP 6: GET PLENTY OF ZZZ'S

Aside from times of stress, consider what other situations generally have you reaching for something sweet. If you're like most of us, cravings tend to occur later in the day, especially when you're starting to feel tired or fatigued. A good night's sleep can keep you from feeling the afternoon blahs. What do you usually find yourself reaching for between 2:00 and 4:00 p.m.? Do you go for another large cup of caffeine (maybe with a hefty dose of sugar in it) or a candy bar, maybe something salty and crunchy made from processed flour? Or has food marketing lulled you into believing that granola bars, date-based bars, and sports bars are a healthy option?

When doing any type of detoxification program, sleep is always a top priority. As we are focusing specifically on sugar, it is important to recognize the abundance of clinical research tying sugar cravings with circadian rhythms and sleep patterns. Too little sleep will trigger a whole lot of sugar cravings. Sleep can be a major make-or-break factor, so take steps ahead of embarking on a sugar detox to improve the quality of your sleep.

Some basic tips to improve sleep:

- Support your natural circadian rhythm through exposure to light and darkness.

- Get some exercise, but not too late in the day.

- Watch your intake: Try not to eat or drink anything (except water) for two to three hours before bed.

- Cut off caffeine by 2 p.m., or noon if you struggle with sleep issues.

- Avoid exposing yourself to anything that may drive nighttime tension or anxiety.

- Develop a bedtime routine at night.

- Set a sleep and wake schedule and stick with it, even on the weekends.

- Adopt a device detox routine. Choose a cutoff time to cease exposure to the blue light and stimulation from electronic devices. Even consider using blue light–blocking glasses. There are clear lens options for daytime use, especially good for those who spend a lot of time in front of screens, and then yellow-tinted lenses to be worn a couple of hours before your intended bedtime.

SUPPORTING DETOXIFICATION PATHWAYS THROUGH FOOD

Before I break down suggestions based on the macronutrient classes of protein, carbohydrates, and fats, a few thoughts. You are aiming to wean off of sugar, not to impose a hard stop of all sources of carbohydrates.

Refer often to your goal-planning tools to help you maintain direction and motivation. Take it day by day, even hour by hour when cravings are trying get the best of you. Write down on a sticky note: "Did I make healthy choices most of the time today?" Stick that note somewhere you will see it each night before you go to bed. Ask and answer the question every night as a means to check in with yourself. If the answer is in the affirmative, great job, you're on the right track. Keep going. If you answer in the negative, brush yourself off, pick yourself up, do not beat yourself up, and with a nonjudgmental heart, ask yourself what happened that day. After you spend a few moments reflecting on what threw you off course, recommit to your program and the prospect that the following night, you will be able to answer with a resounding yes! Give yourself the peace and forgiveness of recognizing that a setback is often a teachable moment, and don't be afraid to seek out the lessons within these moments.

I want to first highlight the foods that are known to support detoxification so that you may begin focusing on these and planning for their routine inclusion in your diet.

- Cruciferous vegetables. Eat at least 1 to 2 cups daily of cabbage, broccoli, bok choy, collards, kale, and Brussels sprouts, as these are rich in sulforaphane, a compound that helps to boost detox in the liver.

- Garlic cloves.

- Decaffeinated green tea. Try to drink it before noon.

- Fresh, whole vegetable juices made with kale, celery, cilantro, beets, parsley, ginger, and small amounts of carrot. Try not to use fruit, but if you must, then use only one serving of fruit to three servings of vegetables.

- Herbal tea such as burdock root, dandelion root, ginger root, licorice root, sarsaparilla root, cardamom seed, or cinnamon (not cassia) bark.

- High-quality, sulfur-containing proteins including eggs or plant protein isolates (with the exception of soy).

- Citrus peels, caraway, and dill oil. These are sources of limonene.

- Antioxidant/bioflavonoid/polyphenol-rich berries, grapes, citrus, and other dark, richly colored fruits.

- Dandelion greens. These can help in liver detoxification by improving the flow of bile and increasing urine flow.

- Celery. This can also increase urine flow.

- Fresh cilantro. To help eliminate heavy metals (not our focus in this detox). By the way, if cilantro tastes like soap to you, it's in your genes—there's a gene variant for that!

- Rosemary. This antioxidant supports expression of detoxification enzyme genes, chelates heavy metals, and promotes anti-inflammatory effects.

- Turmeric/curcuminoids. Also an antioxidant, this supports detoxification and promotes anti-inflammatory effects.

WHAT YOU WON'T SEE ON THE DIET AND WHY

GLUTEN

You won't be seeing gluten-containing grains like wheat, barley, and rye.

You may be familiar with the media-fueled frenzies around gluten-free and grain-free diets, and most detox programs exclude these items because of some specific proteins found in them. Gluten, gliadin, and agglutinin have been shown to be irritating to the lining of the GI tract and increase the likelihood of intestinal permeability. Furthermore, the use of glyphosate (Roundup) prior to harvest of the grains has also been shown to be a contributing factor to the increased prevalence of gluten intolerance. Both intestinal permeability and gluten intolerance have been linked to increasing rates of autoimmune issues, obesity, and other chronic health problems. I would encourage you to consider removing these grains for three to four weeks as part of the detox from sugar in order to allow for greater healing of your GI tract. We are also working under the assumption that you will be dealing with a certain degree of inflammation and potentially increased intestinal permeability just by the nature of your high sugar and refined carbohydrate intake. This does not mean, however, that you should run straight to the store and purchase gluten-free versions of your favorite products. The majority of gluten-free products on the market today are highly processed and can even be higher in carbohydrates and simple sugars than their gluten-containing counterparts. Just like processed, refined wheat products, many gluten-free products also lack fiber and key nutrients and are not recommended.

DAIRY PRODUCTS

Dairy is frequently omitted during detoxification. One reason is the presence of lactose and the prevalence of lactose intolerance. In addition, the composition of dairy proteins, such as casein and whey, are allergens that may trigger other intolerance. Dairy is also considered to be a proinflammatory food group, so if you're looking to maximize power before a detox plan, I'd suggest that you refrain from dairy for the first three to four weeks.

If you choose to remove them from your program for three to four weeks, at some point you may wish to reintroduce those foods. Take some time to note how you have been feeling over the course of the past few weeks off of sugar, dairy, and gluten. You may also want to ask yourself if foods that contain dairy and gluten are also those that may trigger or have an association with your previous consumption of sugar. This may help you to determine whether or not you wish to return gluten and dairy into your diet. If you do decide to bring one or both back, it is worth the time and effort to follow some specifics.

- Don't bring them both back on the same day.
- Choose one food and consume one to two servings of that food over the course of a day.
- The next day, do not consume that food or reintroduce anything else, as this will be your day of watchful waiting. Be mindful of how you feel, literally from head to toe. Any headaches; changes in digestion; pain; fatigue; changes in mood, sleep, focus, or concentration; or food cravings?
- If you don't experience any adverse effect, then on the third day, you can introduce another gluten or dairy food.

I would caution you against falling back into habits where gluten and dairy items take center stage when it comes to your food choices.

HOW LONG DO I NEED TO DETOX?

Contrary to other plans that are based on an ultra-restrictive program for a few days to a few weeks, our plan is meant to provide a gradual release from sugar while reshaping your eating habits with balance for long-term success. If you are someone who prefers finite specifics and limits, then consider following the plan for a minimum of two weeks to an ideal of four weeks, and then moving into long-term dietary and lifestyle change with your new habits taking root and thriving—without sugar. As this is not intended to be a strict elimination program, there is no need to follow a specific reintroduction plan, with the exception of refraining from gluten and dairy as discussed above.

CHOOSING CARBOHYDRATES

You may need to alter these based on your own personal tolerances, but during your sugar detox and beyond, the recommended amount of digestible carbohydrate ranges between 45 and 65 percent of total calories. This number will vary greatly by individual, and personalization is the key to finding the right balance of macronutrients to meet your unique needs.

Minimize and avoid consumption of:

- simple and refined sugars
- artificial and nonnutritive sweeteners as they confuse the brain, trigger cravings, and wreak havoc on the microbiome
- foods made with refined flours (typically white stuff): white breads, white crackers, pretzels, cookies, cakes
- alcohol
- sweetened beverages

Aim for unprocessed or minimally processed complex carbohydrates (remember, the ones referred to as polysaccharides or starches). These carbs will take longer to be digested and absorbed, therefore keeping you fuller longer while also helping to keep blood glucose levels more stable. Vegetables, beans, peas, lentils, and whole grains are included in the complex carbohydrates category. Limit how often you eat starchier foods like potatoes, corn, and white rice. Be sure to aim for the following:

- Whole grain. If you choose not to refrain from gluten and keep all grains in, look for whole grain, which is a step above whole wheat. Don't even bother with any "naked" grains, the white stuff: sugar, white breads, and white flours. The other coverings have been removed in processing, along with fiber and their key nutritional value.

- Get proficient with reading food labels, ingredient lists, and nutrition facts. If you see less than 3 grams of fiber in a grain-based cereal, bread, or cracker, it's likely too processed for our detox purposes. Put it back and choose one with more fiber.

- If you see the term "enriched," especially immediately before a type of flour, that's a red flag to alert you that the flour has been highly processed and the manufacturer tried to replace nutrients that were lost in processing. Put it back and choose another.

- Consume at least 25 to 30 grams of fiber per day.
  - » Soluble fiber. This type of fiber dissolves in water to form a gel-like material. It can help lower blood cholesterol and glucose levels. Soluble fiber is found in oats, peas, beans, apples, citrus fruits, carrots, barley, and psyllium.

  - » Insoluble fiber. This type of fiber promotes the movement of material through your digestive system and increases stool bulk, so it can benefit those who struggle with constipation or irregular stools. Whole-wheat flour, wheat bran, nuts, beans, and vegetables such as cauliflower, green beans, and potatoes are good sources of insoluble fiber.

Boost the detox power of your carb choices and go for the items that don't come packaged or need a nutrition facts label. Stick to the outer-perimeter produce section of your grocery store.

Choose foods that naturally *come from* plants, not foods that *were made in* manufacturing plants!

Don't forget, quality counts! I encourage my clients to opt for organic and non-GMO foods as much as realistically possible for them. I have not seen enough evidence to convince me about the safety of GMO foods, but there is enough research showing the cause for concern and how they may be detrimental to health. Thus, when working toward supporting detoxification successfully, in my opinion, there is no room for GMO foods.

Sugar beets are a top GMO crop from which most commercially available sugar is made. High-fructose corn syrup and other corn-based sweeteners are also manufactured from GMO corn. Oh, and by the way, no fake or Frankenfood foods either—EVER! That means no fake "plant-based burger meats," processed oils, fat substitutes, margarines, spreads, or shortening. Otherwise you'll be impairing detox pathways all over again.

During a sugar detox, the bulk of your carbohydrate intake should be coming from non-starchy vegetables. Try to consume at least five servings (one serving is equivalent to ½ cup cooked or 1 cup raw veggies). Be sure to choose all colors of the rainbow, especially dark leafy greens, dark orange, yellow, and purple. Colorful produce will provide the antioxidants and phytonutrients necessary not only for detoxification but also for overall health. Fruits also provide important nutrients and fiber but will contribute too much sugar if you consume too much. Keep it to one to two servings per day of whole fruits. Eat them; do not drink them.

CHOOSING PROTEINS

Proteins are the construction material for the body. According to current recommendations, a healthy adult human requires 0.8 grams of protein per kilogram of healthy body weight. Ideally, protein should make up about 10 to 15 percent of your total energy intake. Most Americans' diets exceed the recommended amount of protein.

Your protein requirements will increase during times of stress and disease. They are the building blocks for muscles, tissues, neurotransmitters, hormones, enzymes, immune cells, compounds required for detox, etc. Meals with protein also help to balance blood sugar, as do meals with fat, due to the longer digestive process than with carbohydrates alone.

Here are the keys to choosing protein-containing foods during your sugar detox and beyond. You may need to alter these based on your own personal tolerances.

- Remember, quality still counts here too! Consider eating more organic, non-GMO, plant-based protein sources. These include legumes like beans and peas, lentils, spirulina, nutritional yeast, and nuts and seeds. Consider opting for a meatless meal a few times per week to get you comfortable with more plant-based foods and meals. Tofu Tuesdays, anyone?

- If/when you choose to consume animal protein, aim for lean, organic, free-range, grass-fed, wild-caught, or low-mercury as often as possible.

- Eggs (both whites *and* yolks), cheese, poultry, seafood/fish, and even beef and pork are good sources of protein. Just be sure to choose quality sources as described in the previous bullet. (Remember to restrict dairy for a few weeks at first.)

- Dairy products like milk, kefir, and yogurt pull double duty providing protein and carbohydrates. During the first three to four weeks of sugar detoxing I would suggest refraining from dairy and sticking with unsweetened dairy alternatives.

- I repeat, no fake foods! That goes doubly true for the onslaught of plant-based meat substitutes that have hit the market in the last couple of years.

CHOOSING FATS

Fats will provide you with the essential fatty acids, omega-3s and omega-6s, which are a necessary component of brain and heart health. They will also provide anti-inflammatory benefits. Insufficient intakes of omega-3s have been linked to numerous health concerns, such as depression, mood disorders, and cognitive decline. Fats provide flavor and texture and contribute to the feeling of satiety after a meal. Since meals that contain fat and protein take longer to digest and absorb, this also can also help with maintaining balance in blood sugars after meals. Fats are needed for the body to properly absorb the fat-soluble vitamins A, D, E, and K.

Here are the keys to choosing fat-containing foods during your sugar detox and beyond. You may need to alter these based on your own personal tolerances.

- Quality still holds fast, so look for minimally refined, organic, cold-pressed, and non-GMO oils as often as you can.

- After our in-depth discussions, I hope you can let go of the fat fear mongering of the last few decades and stop blaming the butter for what the white bread did! You are now armed with the tools to choose healthy fats.

- Let me say it again: No fake foods, especially fake fats. Let's leave the processed oils, fat substitutes, margarines, spreads, and shortening in the time capsule where they belong and will never rot, alongside the Twinkie and McDonald's fry that's been there for decades. Plus, fake fats are sources of trans fat, which are strongly linked to cardiovascular and brain health issues.

- Wild-caught, low-mercury, cold-water fish is an excellent source of your healthy omega-3 fatty acids. The fish most associated with high levels of mercury include shark, bigeye tuna, swordfish, king mackerel, tilefish, bass, walleye, and pickerel, so choose these less often.

- Choose whole-food natural fats like olives, avocados, coconut, real butter, quality dairy fat (no need for skim/fat-free or 1 percent/low-fat dairy), and nuts or seeds.

- Don't overdo it on saturated fat—lard, cream, butter, fatty cuts of beef, lamb, pork, poultry skin, and cheese.

- Let's just set the record straight on animal fats, especially beef. Quality absolutely does make a difference. The fatty acid profile of conventional beef has a much higher content of omega-6 fatty acids, which are considered to be pro-inflammatory and consumed in excess in the American diet, than grass-fed beef. Grass-fed beef has a more balanced fatty acid profile.

- Be picky, even a little snobbish, with your choice of oils. Familiarize yourself with how the oils smell so you can detect rancid oils. If it fails a sniff test, throw it out. It may be really tempting to buy a large bottle from your local warehouse store, but unless you were going through multiple servings of oil per day for a large family, you run the risk of it going bad before you finish the bottle.

- For cooking oils, personally I prefer heavier, heartier oils such as avocado oil, butter, ghee, virgin coconut oil, and extra-virgin olive oil (EVOO). These are more stable fats and can hold up to higher heat, with the exception of EVOO, which is best for medium, not high, heat.

- Lower-temperature cooking/baking, salad dressings, or cooking where a lighter flavor is desired are best served by lighter and more delicate oils, such as nut or seed oils like almond, flaxseed, grapeseed, hempseed, sesame, sunflower, walnut, etc. If you choose to use safflower or sunflower oils, be sure to use those labeled high-oleic.

MY DETOX TOOLBOX

As we have toured through the macronutrient groups in depth, I hope you now see the link between balancing the consumption of these three groups and maintaining balance in the body. This will be an important factor in your sugar detox, as maintaining an adequate intake of protein and fat can help to lessen some of the cravings and withdrawal symptoms you might experience.

Below you will find a foods map—a cheat sheet of what foods to include and what ones to limit or exclude. In the recipe chapter that follows, there are seventy recipes for you to explore to help you get comfy with your new plan. Since I believe passionately in personalizing nutrition, I find that firm "meal plans" yield little compliance as they rarely reflect personal food preferences, unless they are developed one-on-one with a nutrition provider.

Furthermore, as I want you to focus more on the quality of foods, the balance in your choices, the flavors in your new foods, and how they make you feel, I don't want you to get bogged down with macro ratios, grams of this or that, calories, etc. Therefore, I have opted to exclude the nutritional breakdown of each recipe. I want you to trust in the balance of the recipes provided and not judge things only by numbers—that's how too many people ended up on the diet roller coaster in the first place.

Finally, you'll see a list of twenty tips for success. I hope you have found this journey to be insightful, motivating, and a bit less scary than it seemed in the beginning. I hope you feel ready to break free from the weighing down of sugar addiction. If you need additional support, be sure to seek out a licensed functional nutrition provider in your area. If you're interested in working one-on-one with me or in enrolling in one of my group programs, reach out to me at DrDana.Elia@gmail.com.

DR. DANA'S SUGAR DETOX FOODS CHEAT SHEET

VEGETABLES (5 CUPS/DAY)

INCLUDE		LIMIT
Artichokes	Fermented veggies	Acorn squash
Arugula	Garlic	Butternut squash
Asparagus	Greens, all	Corn
Beets	Horseradish	Plantain
Bok choy	Kale	*Root vegetables:*
Broccoli	Kohlrabi	such as beets,
Broccoli sprouts	Leeks	carrots, parsnips,
Brussels sprouts	Lettuce, all	potatoes, radishes,
Cabbage	Moringa	rutabaga, sweet
Carrots	Mung bean sprouts	potatoes, yams
Cauliflower	Mushrooms	
Celery	Okra	
Chives	Onions	
Chlorella	Peppers	
Cilantro	Radishes	
Cucumbers	Scallions	
Daikon radishes	Sea vegetables	
Dandelion	Shallots	
Eggplant	*Squash:* pumpkin,	
Endive	spaghetti, yellow,	
Escarole	zucchini	
Fennel	Tomato	
	Turnip	

PROTEIN

INCLUDE		AVOID/LIMIT
Eggs	*Protein powder:* egg, hemp, pea, rice, soy protein isolate, whey	All high-mercury fish, such as tuna, shark, swordfish, king mackerel, tilefish, tilapia
Fish: anchovy, halibut, mahi mahi, rainbow trout, salmon, sardines	*Legumes:* black beans, cannellini beans, edamame, garbanzo beans/chickpeas	Bacon
Meat: grass-fed beef, buffalo, elk, pork, lamb, venison, or other wild game	Green lentils	Charbroiled meat
		Fried meat
	Green peas	Grain-fed beef
Poultry: pasture raised, organic	Lima beans	Non-pasture-raised pork
Tofu	Pinto beans	Non-pasture-raised poultry
Tempeh	Red lentils	
Spirulina		

NUTS/SEEDS

INCLUDE		
Almonds	Hazelnuts	Pumpkin seeds
Brazil nuts	Hemp seeds	Sesame seeds
Cashews	Macadamia nuts	Soy nuts
Chia seeds	Pecans	Sunflower seeds
Coconut	Pine nuts	Unsweetened nut/seed butters
Flaxseed	Pistachios	Walnuts

FATS

INCLUDE		AVOID/LIMIT
Choose organic, cold-pressed, non-GMO oils	High-oleic safflower oil	Hydrogenated fats and oils
Avocado oil	High-oleic sunflower oil	Lard
Coconut oil	Sesame oil	Margarine
Extra-virgin olive oil (EVOO)	Walnut oil	Processed fats
Flaxseed oil	Avocados	Shortening
Ghee/clarified butter	Coconut	Trans fats
Grapeseed oil	Olives	
	Butter	
	Coconut milk	

FRUITS (LIMIT 1–2/DAY)

INCLUDE		
Apples	Grapes	Peaches
Apricots	Guavas	Pears
Bananas	Kiwis	Pineapples
Black mulberries	Lemons	Plums
Black raspberries	Mandarins	Pomegranates
Blueberries	Mangoes	Prunes
Cherries	Melons	Raisins
Cranberries	Nectarines	Raspberries
Figs	Oranges	Strawberries
Grapefruits	Papayas	Tangerines

HERBS/SPICES/CONDIMENTS

INCLUDE		
Apple cider vinegar (ACV)	Cumin seeds	Mustard seeds
Balsamic vinegar	Curry	Natural mayo (with olive oil or avocado oil)
Black pepper	Dill	Oregano
Cayenne pepper	Fennel seeds	Organic ketchup
Cinnamon	Garlic	Rosemary
Coriander	Ginger (fresh and ground)	Sea salt
Cumin	Himalayan salt	Turmeric

BEVERAGES

INCLUDE	LIMIT	AVOID
Coconut water	Coffee	Alcohol
Filtered water stored in glass containers/ pitchers	Green tea	Fast food
Kefir (water or coconut kefir)		Fruit juice
Kombucha, no added sweetener (8 ounces max/day)		Soda
Mineral water		Soft drinks
Unsweetened plant milks (coconut, almond, cashew, hemp, flax, hazelnut)		
Herbal teas: chamomile, chicory, dandelion, fennel, hibiscus, honeybush, lavender, nettle, rooibos		

GRAINS (LIMIT 1–2/DAY)

INCLUDE		AVOID
Amaranth	Gluten-free rolled or steel-cut oats	Barley
Brown, black, purple, red, or wild rice	Millet	Corn
Buckwheat	Nut/seed crackers	Rye
	Quinoa	Wheat

DAIRY AND ALTERNATIVES

INCLUDE		AVOID
Unsweetened plant milks (coconut, almond, cashew, hemp, flax, hazelnut)	Unsweetened kefir (soy or coconut)	All other dairy
	Unsweetened cultured yogurt (soy, nut, or coconut)	

DR. DANA'S TOP 20 TIPS FOR SUCCESS

1. Read food labels, ingredient lists, and nutrition facts.

2. Steer clear of all added and refined sugars, especially HFCS.

3. No fake foods.

4. Keep a journal (not just one to log food in).

- Write about your goals and why they are important to you.
- Jot down what you're grateful for.
- Positive affirmations or intentions.
- What's been working well for you, what are you struggling with.

5. Meal plan and meal prep each week. Even if you're going strong, don't scrimp on this habit.

6. Eat more meals prepared at home.

7. Eat adequate protein: 0.8 grams to 1.0 grams per kilogram of body weight.

8. Skip the simple and processed carbohydrates.

9. Examine sources of sugars in your beverages.

10. Make rest and relaxation high priorities. Lack of sleep sets in motion chemical messages in the body that trigger sugar cravings.

11. Develop a daily routine with a wake time, mealtimes, self-care time, and bedtime.

12. Explore integrative self-care practices. Explore even something as simple as deep-breathing exercises or one of the many different forms of meditation.

13. Move your body every day. Make movement and exercise a priority now and for life.

14. Never go grocery shopping without a list, and stick to it.

15. Never shop when you're hungry or tired.

16. No negative self-talk. If you have a slip-up that's okay. It can be a teachable moment to reflect on your goals.

17. Use a buddy system. Partner with a friend, family member, or coworker.

18. Ditch the dried fruit and fruit juices.

19. Go easy with the alcohol.

20. Most of all, remember: "The struggle is part of the journey." So treat yourself with a mindful mind and a nonjudgmental heart.

CHAPTER 8

RECIPES

BREAKFAST

Trifecta Berry Delight

Want to start off the day with a simple and colorful yet sweet and satisfying breakfast? Then look no further. This colorful and eye-appealing bowl is packed with fiber and protein that will keep you going until lunch. Makes a great afternoon snack too.

Prep time: 10 to 12 minutes | *Cook time:* None |
Makes: 2 servings

¾ cup strawberries, sliced

¾ cup blueberries

¾ cup blackberries

2 tablespoons hemp seeds

2 tablespoons chia seeds

¼ cup slivered almonds or pecans

2 tablespoons of your favorite unsweetened nut butter

½ cup unsweetened almond milk

1. Place the berries in a medium bowl.

2. Add the hemp seeds, chia seeds, and slivered almonds and gently mix.

3. Divide the mixture into two serving bowls. I love to use parfait glasses or even a nice mug, so feel free to be creative with the choice of serving dish.

4. Top each bowl with 1 tablespoon of the nut butter.

5. Pour ¼ cup of the almond milk on top of each berry bowl and savor the sweet goodness of antioxidants.

Protein-Powered Banana Pancakes with Berry Topping

Who needs syrups when pureed fruits provide all the necessary sweetness, and cinnamon enhances flavor? Berries are a low-glycemic fruit but pack a lot of flavor and nutrients. You can use whichever berries you have on hand, such as blueberries, raspberries, or strawberries. The protein powder and flaxseed also help to keep you fuller longer.

Prep time: 10 minutes | *Cook time:* 5 minutes | *Makes:* 2 servings

1 egg

¼ cup protein powder, unflavored or vanilla

1 tablespoon ground flaxseed

1 banana, mashed

1 tablespoon unsweetened almond milk

1 teaspoon ground cinnamon, plus more for sprinkling

¼ teaspoon ground nutmeg

¼ cup rolled oats (preferably certified gluten-free)

½ teaspoon organic, cold-pressed, extra-virgin coconut oil

½ cup pureed berries of choice

1. In a large mixing bowl, mix the egg, protein powder, flaxseed, banana, almond milk, cinnamon, nutmeg, and rolled oats.

2. Heat the coconut oil in a large frying pan over medium-low heat.

3. Pour the batter into the pan and cook the pancakes for about 2 to 3 minutes per side. When you see small bubbles forming, the pancakes are stiff enough to flip.

4. Serve with the pureed berries spooned on top and sprinkle the pancakes with the extra cinnamon.

Pumpkin Spice 'n' Everything Nice Overnight Oats

I never need a reason to go for something pumpkin spice, regardless of the season. Every autumn I roast up numerous pumpkins and make my puree to freeze and use throughout the year. Plus, our chickens and dog love pumpkin. It's such a healthy treat for them too. You can make variations of this basic breakfast recipe by swapping out the pumpkin for any other favorite—apples, pears, peaches, etc. Be creative.

Prep time: 15 minutes, plus overnight to chill | *Cook time:* 10 to 12 minutes | *Makes:* 4 servings

1½ cups rolled oats (preferably certified gluten-free)

1½ cups unsweetened almond milk

2 tablespoons chia seeds

1 tablespoon avocado oil

¼ cup pumpkin puree, canned or your own

1 teaspoon ground cinnamon

¼ teaspoon ground nutmeg

¼ teaspoon ground ginger

½ teaspoon vanilla extract

½ cup water

1 cup chopped walnuts or pecans

nut or seed butter of choice, to serve (optional)

1. Combine the rolled oats, almond milk, chia seeds, avocado oil, pumpkin, cinnamon, nutmeg, ginger, vanilla extract, and water in a large glass jar or bowl. Be sure to stir well to evenly mix all the ingredients. Cover tightly and store in the refrigerator overnight.

2. Remove the oat mixture from the refrigerator. Divide the oat mixture into four small oven-safe containers. I like to use glass jars or ramekins. Top each of the jars with ¼ cup of the chopped nuts.

3. Warm the jars in a 350°F oven for 10 to 12 minutes, or if you must, microwave it for 60 seconds.

4. This recipe can be kept in the fridge for 3 to 4 days if you want to make a batch ahead of time or if you have leftovers.

5. If you want to boost the protein content of this breakfast, swirl in some of your favorite unsweetened nut or seed butter.

Mexican Fiesta Omelets

Add a little "funfetti" into your breakfast by choosing color (and phytonutrients) in your omelets with colorful peppers and tomatoes. You can also substitute some fresh salsa in place of the diced tomato. Even a dollop of guac is great on top of this omelet in place of the diced avocado. For the bell pepper, choose red, green, yellow, or orange; the choice is up to you.

Prep time: 10 minutes | *Cook time:* 6 minutes |
Makes: 2 servings

1 tablespoon extra-virgin cold-pressed coconut oil

4 eggs, whisked

¼ cup unsweetened almond milk

½ bell pepper, finely diced

1 cup black beans, cooked, drained, and rinsed, divided

½ cup diced mushrooms

1½ teaspoons chili powder

1 teaspoon ground nutmeg

1 teaspoon paprika

½ avocado, diced

½ medium tomato, diced

sea salt and black pepper, to taste

1. Place the coconut oil in a large frying pan over medium-low heat.

2. Mix the eggs, almond milk, bell pepper, half the black beans, mushrooms, chili powder, nutmeg, and paprika in a large mixing bowl. Beat with a fork.

3. Pour the egg mixture into the frying pan and let cook for about 3 minutes. Fold it in half when the bottom of the omelet firms up and begins to brown. Continue to cook for another 3 minutes.

4. Plate the omelet and top with the diced avocado, tomato, and the remaining black beans. Finish with sea salt and pepper to taste.

Voila Crêpes

You don't need a crêpe machine or crêpe maker for this dish. An 8-inch skillet will work just fine, and you do not need to be a French-trained chef to pull off a great crêpe.

Prep time: 10 minutes | *Cook time:* 15 minutes | *Makes:* 2 servings

1½ tablespoons extra-virgin olive oil, divided

12 cremini or baby bella mushrooms, sliced

3 scallions, chopped

1½ cups spinach

1½ cups endive

2 cloves garlic, minced

½ teaspoon sea salt, divided

¼ cup unsweetened, organic, full-fat coconut milk

3 eggs

½ cup almond flour

½ teaspoon oregano

½ teaspoon nutritional yeast

1. In a large skillet, place three-quarters of your oil and heat over medium-high heat. Add the mushrooms, scallions, spinach, and endive, and sauté until the endive is wilted and the mushrooms have softened.

2. Add the garlic and a pinch of the salt and continue sautéing for 1 more minute.

3. Pour in the coconut milk and stir. Reduce the heat to low to keep warm.

4. In a medium mixing bowl, beat the eggs. Then add the almond flour, oregano, nutritional yeast, and the rest of the salt and mix very well.

5. Add just enough oil to coat the bottom of an 8-inch pan, and place it on the stovetop over medium heat.

6. Holding the pan on an angle, pour ¼ cup of the crêpe batter into the pan and with a rotating wrist, move the pan swiftly in a circle to allow the batter to evenly coat the pan.

7. Cook for 60 to 90 seconds, watching closely for when the crêpe becomes slightly golden brown around the edges and lifts easily from the pan. Flip the crêpe over and continue cooking for another 30 to 60 seconds. Repeat this process until you cook all of the batter, adding more oil to the pan as needed.

8. Plate the crêpe, drop a spoonful of the mushroom filling into the middle of the crêpe, and then fold or roll.

Cauliflower Eggy Bites

Eggs are one of nature's perfect foods. We raise our own hens, so there's never a shortage of eggs in my house. Having breakfast options that travel well and are portable also helps to ensure you stay on track. These egg bites are muffin-sized, and two will count as 1 serving. Make these over the weekend to have a quick and easy breakfast or lunch during the week. They will easily reheat in a toaster oven (or a microwave if you must).

Prep time: 10 minutes | *Cook time:* 15 minutes |
Makes: 6 servings

5 cups cauliflower rice

6 eggs

1 cup spinach, roughly chopped

½ cup asparagus, chopped

¼ cup carrot, finely chopped

¼ cup parsley, finely chopped

½ cup nutritional yeast

sea salt and black pepper, to taste

1. Preheat the oven to 375°F. Prepare your muffin pan with paper liners or by lightly greasing each well with oil or cooking spray.

2. Add the cauliflower rice, eggs, spinach, asparagus, carrot, parsley, nutritional yeast, sea salt, and pepper to a large mixing bowl. Mix well to combine.

3. Using a ¼ cup scooper, scoop the mix into each well of the muffin pan. Place the muffin pan in the oven and bake for 15 minutes.

4. Remove the eggy bites from the oven and allow them to cool for a few minutes to set before popping the bites from each well. Store in the fridge.

A Real Wonder Bread

When searching for a good bread recipe to satisfy cravings, look no further! If you prefer savory bread, add some onion, garlic, rosemary, or thyme. For a dessert, opt for pumpkin spices or cinnamon. Let your creative juices flow with the basic bread recipe that's full of fiber, protein, and healthy fat while also providing a lower-carb option for bread lovers. Toast this up for sandwiches too. Golden flaxseed meal will give your bread a lighter color, but brown is more widely available.

Prep time: 10 minutes | *Cook time:* 50 minutes | *Makes:* 10 servings

2 cups flaxseed meal

1 tablespoon baking powder

¾ teaspoon sea salt

1 tablespoon everything bagel seasoning, divided

5 room-temperature eggs

½ cup room-temperature water

⅓ cup coconut oil, melted

1½ teaspoons nutritional yeast

1. Preheat the oven to 350°F. Prepare a loaf pan by lightly greasing the inside with a bit of coconut oil or lining it with parchment paper.

2. In a medium mixing bowl, combine the flaxseed meal, baking powder, salt, and half of the everything bagel seasoning. Stir well with a spatula or firm whisk until fully combined.

3. In a small mixing bowl, beat the eggs for 30 to 60 seconds. Add in the water and coconut oil, whisking well until fully combined.

4. Pour the wet ingredients into the bowl of the dry ingredients, and stir well. Let the batter rest for a couple of minutes to allow it to thicken up a bit.

5. Pour the batter into the greased loaf pan and shake it or tap it on the counter to evenly distribute the batter. Place the pan in the oven and bake for about 50 minutes. The bread is done when the top of the loaf appears set and browned.

6. As soon as you remove the loaf from the oven, sprinkle the nutritional yeast and the remaining bagel seasoning on top.

7. Allow the loaf to cool before slicing. Store any leftovers in the fridge for 3 to 4 days or pop it in the freezer for long-term storage.

A Real Wonder Avocado Toast

A quick snack anytime of the day! Toss on a fried egg or two for a meal.

Prep time: 5 minutes | *Cook time:* None |
Makes: 2 servings

2 slices A Real Wonder Bread
(page 157)

½ avocado, mashed

½ tomato, diced

¼ teaspoon sesame seeds

¼ teaspoon extra-virgin olive oil

sea salt, black pepper, and
nutritional yeast, to taste

1. Place two slices of your homemade A Real Wonder Bread in the toaster and toast to your preference.

2. Spread the mashed avocado on the slices of toasted bread.

3. Add the diced tomato and sesame seeds, and drizzle the olive oil on top.

4. Season with sea salt, black pepper, and nutritional yeast to taste and serve.

Southwest Breakfast Skillet

What better way to start off your day than with a swift kick in the flavor department with this breakfast skillet? But who says breakfast recipes can only be eaten for breakfast? This makes a great dinner as well. If cilantro tastes like soap to you, as it does me, feel free to omit it. You can thank your genes for that too.

Prep time: 15 minutes | *Cook time:* 15 minutes | *Makes:* 4 servings

1 tablespoon extra-virgin olive oil

1 pound extra-lean ground beef

½ cup chopped red or yellow onion

2 tablespoons chili powder

1 tablespoon cumin

¼ teaspoon onion powder

¼ teaspoon black pepper

½ cup black beans, rinsed and drained

¼ cup nutritional yeast

4 eggs

½ tomato, chopped

¼ cup black olives

½ avocado, cubed

1 jalapeno pepper, sliced

¼ cup cilantro

1. Heat the olive oil in a large skillet over medium heat. Sauté the ground beef and onion for 10 to 12 minutes or until the beef is completely cooked.

2. Toss in the chili powder, cumin, onion powder, black pepper, beans, and nutritional yeast and stir to combine. Make four wells in the mixture and crack 1 egg into each well.

3. Cover the pan with a lid for 3 minutes or until the yolk sets to your preferred firmness.

4. Remove the skillet from the stove and add the remaining ingredients on top of the meat and eggs.

5. Quarter and serve.

ABC Eggy Crêpes

Who needs breads or wraps when an egg batter can create the perfect crêpe for you to wrap your "sandwich" fixins' in?

Prep time: 10 minutes | *Cook time:* 5 minutes | *Makes:* 4 servings

4 eggs

¼ teaspoon sea salt, plus more to taste

1 teaspoon extra-virgin olive oil, divided

4 large romaine lettuce leaves

8 ounces cooked chicken breast, sliced into thin strips

4 ounces broccoli sprouts

1 tomato, sliced

1 avocado, sliced

mayo (optional)

black pepper, to taste

1. Add the eggs and salt to a medium mixing bowl and whisk.

2. Lightly coat the bottom of an 8-inch pan with oil and heat over medium heat.

3. Holding the pan at an angle, pour ¼ cup of the egg batter into the oiled pan and rotate the pan swiftly to evenly coat the pan with the batter. Cook for 60 to 90 seconds, watching closely for when the crêpe becomes slightly golden brown around the edges and lifts easily from the pan.

4. Flip the crêpe over and continue cooking for another 30 to 60 seconds, then plate. Repeat this process with the remaining batter, adding more oil to the pan as needed.

5. To assemble, lay each crêpe on a serving plate, then add the lettuce, chicken, broccoli sprouts, and tomato and top with the sliced avocado. Season to taste with mayo, salt, and pepper, and serve.

Berry Blast Detox Smoothie

Smoothies are the perfect way to sneak in some veggies at breakfast! Keeping a bag of frozen organic berries on hand at all times makes smoothies simple and quick to whip up anytime. The sweet taste of the berries also helps to balance the greens.

Prep time: 5 minutes | *Cook time:* None | *Makes:* 2 servings

1 tablespoon avocado oil

1 cup frozen blueberries

1 cup frozen raspberries

1 cup baby spinach

1 cup baby kale

2 tablespoons chia seeds

1 scoop protein powder, unflavored or vanilla

1½ cups unsweetened almond milk

1 teaspoon ground cinnamon, plus more to serve

¼ teaspoon vanilla extract

1. Add all of your ingredients to a blender or food processor. Puree until your desired consistency is reached. Pour into serving glasses and sprinkle a bit more cinnamon on top to serve.

Supercharged Smoothie

The green smoothie packs a punch of antioxidants with just the right balance of sweet, tart, and ZING!

Prep time: 10 minutes | *Cook time:* None | *Makes:* 2 servings

4 cups roughly chopped kale

1 cucumber, roughly chopped

juice of 1 lemon

2 green apples, peeled, cored, and roughly chopped

1 scoop protein powder, unflavored or vanilla

1 tablespoon grated ginger

2 teaspoons ground cinnamon, plus more to serve

1 tablespoon ground flaxseed or chia seeds

1½ cups filtered water

½ cup ice cubes

1. Add all of your ingredients to a blender or food processor. Puree until your desired consistency is reached. Pour into serving glasses and sprinkle a bit more cinnamon on top to serve.

APPETIZERS

Adult Ants on a Log

Who says we have to grow up and can't play with our food? If you're not a fan of celery, slices of cucumber can also work.

Prep time: 10 minutes | *Cook time:* None |
Makes: 4 servings

8 stalks celery

½ cup sunflower seed butter or any nut/seed butter of your choice

1 tablespoon chia seeds

1. Slice the celery into 16 sticks, or logs.

2. Spread 1 tablespoon of the nut or seed butter across each celery log.

3. Sprinkle the chia seeds over the logs.

Hummus Coins

Yes, I do like to play with my food, and having finger foods is a great way to deal with snacky cravings. Another good veggie to use for this recipe is daikon radish.

Prep time: 10 minutes | *Cook time:* None | *Makes:* 4 servings

½ cucumber, sliced into rounds

½ yellow or green zucchini, sliced into rounds

½ of a wide carrot, sliced into rounds

1 cup hummus

1 tablespoon everything bagel seasoning

1. Lay the cucumber, zucchini, and carrot slices on a large platter.

2. Place a teaspoonful of hummus onto each slice.

3. Sprinkle the everything bagel seasoning on top of the hummus.

Buffalo Cauliflower Bites

You don't have to give up your favorite foods, but tasty substitutions can make living a healthier lifestyle easier and more realistic for the long-term. If you don't want a breaded option, skip the flours and water.

Prep time: 15 minutes | *Cook time:* 20 to 25 minutes | *Makes:* 4 servings

½ cup almond flour

½ cup coconut flour

1 cup water

1 teaspoon sea salt, plus more to taste

1 teaspoon garlic powder

1 teaspoon onion powder

1 head cauliflower, chopped

3 tablespoons extra-virgin olive oil

½ cup buffalo sauce or hot sauce

black pepper, to taste

1. Preheat the oven to 450°F. Line a baking sheet with parchment paper.

2. In a large mixing bowl, combine the flours, water, salt, and garlic and onion powders. Whisk together until smooth.

3. Place the cauliflower into the batter and toss until the cauliflower is evenly coated.

4. Place the cauliflower on the baking sheet, making sure not to overlap pieces.

5. Place the pan in the oven and bake for 15 to 20 minutes, or until the cauliflower is lightly browned.

6. In a small bowl, mix the olive oil with the buffalo or hot sauce and pour evenly over the cauliflower pieces.

7. Bake for 5 minutes, turn the bites over, and bake for 5 minutes more.

8. Season with sea salt and black pepper to taste, and serve.

Balsamic Herbed Mushrooms

Mushrooms are nutrient powerhouses, packed full of B vitamins, vitamin D, selenium, potassium, copper, iron, and phosphorus. Here's a quick, easy recipe to help you increase your mushroom intake. Cooked or raw, white, button, baby bella, or cremini—the sky is the limit for these gems. One of the things I love most about cooking with balsamic vinegar is the fact that the vinegar caramelizes and adds a sweetness without all the sugar and calories. This also tastes great as a topping over burgers, steaks, or chops.

Prep time: 10 minutes | *Cook time:* 8 to 10 minutes | *Makes:* 2 servings

5 cups halved mushrooms

2 tablespoons balsamic vinegar

2 teaspoons Italian seasoning or herbes de Provence

1 teaspoon extra-virgin olive oil

2 cloves garlic, minced

1 shallot, chopped

1. Place all of the ingredients in a large skillet over medium-high heat.

2. Sauté for 8 to 10 minutes. The mushroom volume will reduce, and they will become tender. Allow the vinegar to thicken as it caramelizes.

3. Remove from the heat and enjoy.

"Bet You Can't Eat Just One" Kale Chips

Who wouldn't go crazy for these yummy snacks? They don't last long in my house. You can create any number of flavor variations by swapping out the herbs and spices for your favorites. Instead of onion and garlic powder, use cinnamon and nutmeg; rosemary and thyme with sea salt; or dill and ranch seasoning. Olive oil works well with savory seasonings, and coconut oil goes better with a "sweeter" flavor profile. You can even swap out the kale for thinly sliced zucchini, daikon radish, or even beets. Be sure to thinly slice any other veggie you try to use.

Prep time: 10 minutes | *Cook time:* 10 to 15 minutes |
Makes: 4 servings

8 cups kale leaves, torn into large pieces

2 tablespoons extra-virgin olive oil

1 teaspoon garlic powder

1 teaspoon onion powder

¼ teaspoon sea salt

1. Preheat the oven to 275°F.

2. Add the kale leaves, olive oil, and seasonings to a large mixing bowl place. With clean hands, mix all the ingredients, massaging the kale leaves to thoroughly coat them.

3. Pour the mixture onto a baking sheet and spread the kale leaves evenly. You do not want to overcrowd the kale leaves or they will steam and get soggy rather than crisp up. You may need to cook them in batches depending on the size of your baking sheet.

4. Place the baking sheet in the oven and bake for 10 to 15 minutes or until the kale is crispy. Watch the oven closely so they don't burn.

5. Remove from the oven and devour!

Tuna-Stuffed Bell Pepper

This is the perfect lunch or light dinner. Flavor it to your preference with any combo of spices. I prefer the everything bagel seasoning or onions and garlic. I will often make a "tuna melt" with this recipe as well, adding a small pinch of grated cheese and placing the peppers in the toaster oven for a minute or two to melt the cheese.

Prep time: 10 minutes | *Cook time:* None |
Makes: 2 servings

1 avocado, mashed

2 tablespoons extra-virgin olive oil

1 teaspoon lemon juice

1 (5- to 6-ounce) can or pouch tuna or salmon

2 bell peppers, halved and deseeded

½ tablespoon nutritional yeast

sea salt and black pepper, to taste

1. In a medium bowl, mash the avocado and mix it well with the olive oil and lemon juice to create a mayo-like spread.

2. Fold in the tuna or salmon.

3. Stuff the pepper halves with your tuna salad.

4. Sprinkle the nutritional yeast on top of each stuffed pepper.

5. Season with sea salt and black pepper to taste, and serve.

Green Bean Almondine

You don't have to wait for a holiday to enjoy some dressed-up green beans.

Prep time: 5 minutes | *Cook time:* 20 minutes | *Makes:* 3 servings

1 pound green beans, trimmed

2 shallots, chopped

2 cloves garlic, minced

2 tablespoons tamari or coconut aminos

2½ tablespoons sesame oil

2 tablespoons sesame seeds

¼ cup slivered almonds

sea salt and black pepper, to taste

1. Preheat the oven to 400°F and line a baking sheet with parchment paper.

2. In a large mixing bowl, combine the green beans, shallots, garlic, tamari, sesame oil, and sesame seeds. Toss well to evenly coat the beans.

3. Pour the mixture onto the baking sheet and give it a shake to spread everything out evenly. Place the sheet in the oven for 10 minutes.

4. Add the almonds, and mix. Bake for an additional 10 minutes.

5. Remove from oven, season with sea salt and black pepper to taste, and serve.

Oven-Fried Jicama Fries

Who doesn't like a good fry every once and while? We're using jicama, but you can easily swap it out for zucchini or even eggplant. Just cut the baking time down to about 15 to 20 minutes for them. This recipe would be a great side for the Not Your Nana's Meatloaves or even the OPA! Burgers.

Prep time: 10 minutes | *Cook time:* 50 minutes |
Makes: 4 servings

1 large jicama, sliced into fries

1 tablespoon extra-virgin olive oil

¼ teaspoon paprika

¼ teaspoon garlic powder

¼ teaspoon onion powder

¼ teaspoon herbes de Provence

½ teaspoon sea salt

1. Preheat the oven to 425°F. Line a baking sheet with a sheet of parchment paper.

2. Place the jicama in a large saucepan and cover it with water. Cover and heat on the stovetop over medium-high heat. Bring to a boil, uncover, and cook for 10 minutes. Drain well and place in a large mixing bowl.

3. Add the remaining ingredients and mix well.

4. Lay the fries onto the baking sheet and place it in the oven. Bake for 20 minutes, turn them over, and bake for another 20 minutes.

5. Remove from oven, season with salt and pepper to taste, and dig in.

Oven-Roasted Brussels Sprouts with Walnuts

One of my greatest vegetable regrets is not being exposed to Brussels sprouts early enough in life. Unfortunately, my parents and grandparents were not fans of this wonderful vegetable, so I was not exposed to it until my early twenties, when it was love at first bite. Many people are turned off by Brussels sprouts, either because of their sulfurous smell or because they haven't yet experienced them properly prepared. On holidays, I love to cook them on the stalk, and what a wonderful edible centerpiece they become. They are so simple yet so incredibly healthy. You can use this recipe in your toaster oven or even cook them on the stovetop in a cast-iron skillet or nonstick pan. However you choose to cook them, I hope you learn to love them as much as I do.

Prep time: 5 minutes | *Cook time:* 15 minutes | *Makes:* 4 servings

4 cups Brussels sprouts, trimmed, thinly sliced

3 tablespoons avocado oil

1 tablespoon balsamic vinegar

½ teaspoon garlic powder

½ cup walnuts, chopped

½ teaspoon sea salt

1. Preheat the oven to 375°F. Line a baking sheet with parchment paper.

2. In a large mixing bowl, combine all of the ingredients and toss well.

3. Pour the contents of the bowl onto the baking sheet and shake to spread all the Brussels sprouts and nuts evenly.

4. Place the pan in the oven and roast for 15 minutes or until the sprouts are lightly browned and fork-tender.

5. Serve with your desired protein.

Simply Sinful Chickpeas

We all need a crunchy snack from time to time, and these little balls of deliciousness are packed with protein and fiber to keep you full and satisfied without the guilt. These chickpeas travel well, so keep them on hand for when hunger or a snack craving hits. Modify the recipe to suit the flavors you are most drawn to. Swap out the cinnamon and nutmeg for onion powder, garlic powder, or everything bagel seasoning.

Prep time: 5 minutes | *Cook time:* 60 to 65 minutes | *Makes:* 4 servings

2 cups chickpeas cooked, drained, rinsed, and thoroughly dried

2 tablespoons extra-virgin olive oil or coconut oil, divided

1 teaspoon ground nutmeg

1 teaspoon ground cinnamon

1. Preheat the oven to 350°F. Line a sheet pan with parchment paper.

2. In a medium mixing bowl, combine the dry chickpeas with 1 tablespoon of oil. Stir until the chickpeas are thoroughly coated. Pour the chickpeas onto your baking sheet and spread them apart evenly. Place the sheet in your oven and bake for 25 minutes, then stir the chickpeas and bake for an additional 25 minutes.

3. Remove the baking sheet from oven and place the roasted chickpeas back into your mixing bowl. Pour in the remaining oil, nutmeg, and cinnamon. Stir well to make sure the chickpeas are evenly coated.

4. Return the chickpeas to the baking sheet and bake for another 10 to 15 minutes.

5. Cool the chickpeas for a few minutes before serving. Try not to eat them all in one sitting.

Oven-Roasted Root Veggies

While you want to limit how often you are eating starchier vegetables, they are still full of nutrients and can be a part of your detox plan when playing a supporting role to the leading nonstarchy veggies. So if you're craving potatoes, these oven-roasted root veggies can be a perfect substitute. Packed full of fiber and nutrients but with fewer carbohydrates than potatoes, radishes, especially, taste somewhat sweet when roasted.

Prep time: 15 to 20 minutes | *Cook time:* 20 to 25 minutes | *Makes:* 6 servings

1 cup radishes, trimmed and sliced

1 cup sliced beets

1 cup sliced jicama

2 tablespoons avocado or olive oil

½ teaspoon sea salt

1 teaspoon onion powder

1 teaspoon paprika

1. Preheat the oven to 400°F. Line a large baking sheet with aluminum foil or parchment paper.

2. In a large mixing bowl, combine the veggies with the oil and seasonings. Mix well to ensure all the veggies are well coated.

3. Pour the seasoned veggie mix onto the baking sheet and bake for 20 to 25 minutes, or until the veggies are lightly browned and fork-tender.

4. Add additional seasonings to taste, or toss a bit of balsamic vinegar on top. Serve warm.

Roasted Red Pepper Lentil Hummus

If you like hummus, chickpeas aren't the only option to make a nice dip for your veggies. Lentils and even edamame will blend up quite well to give you a variety of options.

Prep time: 10 minutes | *Cook time:* 15 minutes |
Makes: 6 servings

½ cup dry red lentils, rinsed well

2 cups organic vegetable broth

½ cup roasted red peppers, diced

1½ tablespoons extra-virgin olive oil

1 tablespoon tahini

1 small clove garlic, minced

½ teaspoon onion powder

2 tablespoons lemon juice

¼ teaspoon sea salt

black pepper, to taste

2 tablespoons chopped nuts, such as pine nuts or pistachios

1. Add the lentils and vegetable broth to a medium saucepan over medium heat. Bring the liquid to a low simmer and allow the lentils to cook for 12 to 15 minutes. Once they are tender, remove from the heat and drain well in a mesh strainer.

2. Transfer the lentils to a food processor or blender. Add the peppers, oil, tahini, garlic, onion powder, lemon juice, and salt and puree until the mixture becomes smooth. Add additional salt, pepper, and lemon juice to taste.

3. Place the mixture in a storage container and chill in the fridge for a few hours to overnight.

4. When ready to eat, top with the chopped nuts and serve with sliced raw veggies.

Curry-Roasted Edamame

Edamame makes a great snack that travels well. Feel free to swap out the curry powder for any other seasoning that strikes your fancy—ranch, onion, garlic, or cinnamon. Stick with the extra-virgin olive oil if going with a savory spice palette. Use extra-virgin coconut oil if going with more dessert-type flavors.

Prep time: 5 minutes | *Cook time:* 40 minutes | *Makes:* 2 servings

2 cups shelled edamame

1 tablespoon extra-virgin olive oil

1 teaspoon sea salt

1 teaspoon curry powder

1. Preheat the oven to 375°F. Line a baking sheet with parchment paper.

2. Add all of the ingredients to a large mixing bowl and stir well to coat.

3. Pour the coated edamame out onto a baking sheet and roast in the oven for 20 minutes. Shake the tray to stir up the edamame, and roast for another 20 minutes.

4. Remove from oven, allow to cool for a few minutes, and happy crunching!

Flavor-Forward
Stuffed Avocados

This recipe is both colorful and flavorful. Healthy fats and proteins abound in this dish. You can serve this as an appetizer, side dish, or even the main event. Enjoy!

Prep time: 10 minutes | *Cook time:* None |
Makes: 6 servings

3 large avocados, halved

lemon wedge, plus 1 tablespoon lemon juice

1 tablespoon olive oil

2 tablespoons canned black beans, rinsed

⅓ cup diced cucumber

⅓ cup diced bell pepper

6 tablespoons cherry tomatoes, quartered

½ small red onion, diced

1 clove garlic, minced

2 tablespoons hummus

¼ teaspoon ground sumac

sea salt and black pepper, to taste

nutritional yeast, to taste

1. Place your avocado halves on a serving platter. Scoop a bit more of the flesh out to create a larger space for your stuffing, and place the scooped flesh into a medium mixing bowl. Rub a little bit of lemon juice from the lemon wedge on the flesh of each half to keep the avocado from turning brown.

2. Combine the remaining ingredients in the bowl with the scooped avocado flesh.

3. Spoon the mixture into the wells of the avocados.

4. Season with salt and pepper to taste, adding a bit of nutritional yeast for a cheesy flavor, as desired, and serve.

LUNCH

OPA! Burgers

Now don't go around smashing plates on the kitchen floor! This basic burger recipe can be transformed into meatballs or even into a meatloaf. You can also swap out grass-fed organic beef for the chicken. Stuff these burgers into large portobello mushroom caps and bake them at 350°F for about 30 minutes. Have fun! If you are dairy-free, use nutritional yeast in place of the Parmesan cheese and cashew cheese or tofu in place of the feta.

Prep time: 20 minutes | *Cook time:* 20 minutes |
Makes: 6 servings

2½ teaspoons extra-virgin olive oil, plus more to drizzle

½ cup diced red onion, divided

½ zucchini, diced

1 red bell pepper, diced, divided

4 cups baby spinach

½ cup almond flour

½ cup coconut flour

1 pound extra-lean ground chicken

1 tablespoon grated Parmesan cheese

½ cup crumbled feta cheese, crumbled

½ cup chopped black or green Greek olives, divided

½ cucumber, diced

½ tomato, diced

sea salt and black pepper, to taste

2 cups spring mix greens

2 cups arugula

1. Heat the olive oil in a large skillet over medium heat.

2. Place half of the red onion, zucchini, and red pepper into the skillet and sauté until the onion becomes translucent, about five minutes.

3. Once the onion becomes translucent, add the baby spinach and sauté for an additional 1½ minutes. Turn off the heat and set the pan of veggies aside to cool.

4. In a large mixing bowl, combine the almond flour, coconut flour, chicken, Parmesan cheese, half of the feta cheese, and half of the olives.

5. Once the vegetables from the skillet are cool to the touch, add them to the mixing bowl and mix well with your hands. You will get messy!

6. Roll the mixture into 6 even balls. Flatten the balls into patties and place them on a large baking sheet.

7. Time to fire up your grill to medium heat! (Or, use the large skillet from earlier if cooking indoors).

8. While the grill is heating, prepare the OPA! salsa by mixing the remaining red onion, zucchini, red peppers, and black olives with the feta cheese, cucumber, and tomato, in a small bowl. Coat with a drizzle of extra-virgin olive oil and toss. Season it with sea salt and pepper to taste. Set aside.

9. Add the burgers to the grill or skillet and cook for 7 to 8 minutes per side or until the burgers are cooked through.

10. While the burgers cook, combine the spring mix and arugula in a large bowl.

11. Place each burger over a bed of the combined greens. Add a scoop of the OPA! salsa to each and serve.

Oh So Simple, Zesty Zucchini Spinach Caprese Salad

This classic salad with a twist includes some detox rock stars. You can make this a light lunch or a side salad. For a main event, try adding some grilled chicken, grilled salmon, or grilled shrimp on top. If staying dairy-free, use tofu in place of the mozzarella.

Prep time: 10 to 20 minutes | *Cook time:* None |
Makes: 2 servings

2 zucchini, chopped

2 cups baby spinach

½ cup fresh broccoli florets

1 cup halved cherry tomatoes

juice of 1 lemon

1½ tablespoons balsamic vinegar

2 tablespoons extra-virgin olive oil

1 clove garlic, minced

3.5 ounces fresh mozzarella cheese or bocconcini balls, chopped

½ cup chopped fresh basil leaves

1 teaspoon dried oregano

sea salt and black pepper, to taste

1. Place the zucchini, spinach, broccoli, and cherry tomatoes in a large bowl.

2. In a small bowl or jar, combine the lemon, vinegar, olive oil, and garlic. Whisk or shake well.

3. Add all of the dressing to the large bowl of veggies and mix well.

4. If you're not in a rush to devour this salad, let the dressed veggies marinate in the refrigerator for about 10 minutes.

5. When you are ready to eat, divide the salad between two serving bowls and add the mozzarella, basil, and oregano on top.

6. Season with salt and pepper.

Simple Salmon Salad Lettuce Wraps

Quick to make but big on flavor! Another thing I love to do with tuna, salmon, or chicken salad is to stuff it into a bell pepper instead of lettuce, sprinkle some nutritional yeast on top, and pop it in the toaster oven for a few minutes—yummo.

Prep time: 15 minutes | *Cook time:* None | *Makes:* 2 servings

1 avocado

2 tablespoons lemon juice

1 tablespoon extra-virgin olive oil

¼ teaspoon sea salt

1 (5- to 6-ounce) can or pouch salmon, drained

2 teaspoons everything bagel seasoning

2 scallions, chopped

⅛ cucumber, deseeded and finely chopped

4 leaves romaine lettuce

¼ cup diced tomato

pinch of fresh or dried dill

1. Mash the avocado in a medium mixing bowl, then add the lemon juice, olive oil, and salt to create a mayo-like spread.

2. Stir in the salmon, everything bagel seasoning, scallions, and cucumber. Season with additional salt and pepper if needed.

3. Place 2 romaine leaves on each of two serving plates. Divide the salmon salad evenly between them. Top with the diced tomato and dill and serve!

Curry Quinoa, Carrot, and Kale Cakes

Best served over a bed of your favorite salad greens, these are a meal all by themselves because of the protein content quinoa provides. As a side, pair them with a protein of choice, such as a nice piece of grilled salmon.

Prep time: 15 minutes | *Cook time:* 25 minutes | *Makes:* 6 cakes

½ cup quinoa

1 cup organic vegetable broth

1 tablespoon coconut oil, divided

½ sweet onion, diced

2 cups kale leaves

½ cup finely chopped carrot

2 eggs

3 cloves garlic, minced

1½ teaspoons curry powder

1 tablespoon nutritional yeast

1 tablespoon yellow mustard

½ cup almond flour

sea salt and black pepper, to taste

1. Add the quinoa and broth to a medium saucepan over medium-high heat and bring to a boil. Once boiling, cover, reduce the heat to low, and simmer for 12 minutes. Remove from the heat and fluff with a fork. Set aside.

2. In a large skillet, heat half of the coconut oil over medium heat. Add the onion and sauté until translucent. Toss in the kale and carrot and sauté for 2 to 3 more minutes. Remove from the heat.

3. In a large mixing bowl, beat the eggs. Fold in the quinoa, kale and carrot mixture, garlic, salt, and pepper. Mix well.

4. When the mixture has cooled, add in the curry powder, nutritional yeast, mustard, and almond flour. Mix thoroughly.

5. Divide the mixture into 6 balls. Flatten each ball into the shape of a patty, or cake, and place them on a plate.

6. In the same large skillet, heat the remaining coconut oil over medium heat. When the oil is heated, transfer the quinoa cakes to the skillet and cook until golden brown, 6 to 7 minutes per side.

Dr. Dana's Kickin' Chicken Salad

If you like to pick up a rotisserie chicken every now and then, this is a great salad to make using the leftover chicken. Otherwise just use some cooked chicken breast.

Prep time: 10 minutes | *Cook time:* None |
Makes: 2 servings

1 small onion, finely chopped

1 clove garlic, minced

1 avocado, mashed

1 tablespoon Dijon mustard

1 teaspoon Sriracha chili sauce (or more if you like it hot)

1 teaspoon curry powder

juice of ¼ lemon

3 tablespoons extra-virgin olive oil, divided

6 ounces cooked chicken (white meat preferred), shredded or cubed

3 cups kale leaves, finely chopped

1½ teaspoons hemp seeds

sea salt and black pepper, to taste

1. In a medium mixing bowl, mix the onion, garlic, mashed avocado, mustard, Sriracha sauce, curry powder, lemon juice, and 2 tablespoons of the olive oil. Mix well until a mayo-like consistency forms. Add extra olive oil if needed.

2. Add the chicken to the bowl and combine well.

3. In a separate small bowl, combine the kale and hemp seeds with the remaining olive oil. Season with salt and pepper.

4. Divide the kale between two serving bowls. Add half of the kickin' chicken salad on top of each bowl.

5. Season with additional salt and pepper.

Easy Dreamy Cauliflower Soup

Whether it's a cold night or a lazy afternoon, this quick, simple soup will nourish you, body and soul.

Prep time: 15 minutes | *Cook time:* 45 minutes |
Makes: 4 servings

2 tablespoons extra-virgin olive oil

½ yellow onion, chopped

2 cloves garlic, minced

1 carrot, chopped

1 large head cauliflower, sliced to florets

3 cups organic broth (vegetable or chicken is fine)

1 cup unsweetened, organic coconut milk

¼ teaspoon sea salt

¼ teaspoon black pepper

1 teaspoon ground nutmeg

2 scallions, chopped

1 teaspoon nutritional yeast (optional, to add a cheesy flavor)

1. In a large pot over medium heat, heat the olive oil. Sauté the onion, garlic, and carrot for 5 minutes or until the onion is soft and golden.

2. Add the cauliflower to the pot and cook until it begins to brown, about 5 minutes.

3. Pour the broth into the pot and bring it to a boil. Lower the heat, cover, and let simmer for 30 minutes.

4. Add the coconut milk, sea salt, pepper, and nutmeg. Stir until the coconut milk is fully dispersed and heated through, about 1 to 2 minutes.

5. Transfer the soup to a blender, then puree to a smooth consistency.

6. Pour the soup into your favorite bowl or mug and top with chopped scallions, then sprinkle with nutritional yeast, salt, and pepper to taste.

Bruschetta Tor-Pizzas

One of the biggest challenges for people who are trying to follow a healthier diet is giving up some of their favorite foods—especially comfort foods like pizza. This recipe gives you the flavor and feel of pizza without all the extra calories. Nutritional yeast gives you the flavor of cheese while providing a dairy-free option.

Prep time: 15 minutes | *Cook time:* 15 minutes | *Makes:* 4 servings

4 Roma tomatoes, finely diced

¼ cup sliced black olives

3 cloves garlic, minced

½ cup basil leaves, chopped

1 tablespoon balsamic vinegar

2 tablespoons extra-virgin olive oil

½ cup nutritional yeast

4 brown rice tortillas

4 ounces cooked chicken breast, diced

sea salt and black pepper, to taste

1. Preheat the oven to 400°F. Line a baking pan with aluminum foil.

2. In a large mixing bowl, toss the tomatoes, olives, garlic, basil, vinegar, olive oil, nutritional yeast, salt, and pepper. Pour the mixture into a fine-mesh strainer to drain the extra liquid.

3. Place the tortillas on the lined baking pan. Spoon the vegetables onto the tortillas. Place the chicken on top of the veggies.

4. Bake for 15 minutes, then remove from the oven. Allow to cool for 1 to 2 minutes before slicing and serving.

Tricolor Chicken Mango Quinoa Bowl

This recipe works well, not only with chicken but also with a good-quality substitute like ground turkey. Your other option would be to prepare the quinoa by itself and serve with a mild white fish like mahi mahi or an organic pastured pork loin.

Prep time: 10 minutes | *Cook time:* 30 minutes |
Makes: 4 servings

½ cup quinoa

1 cup organic vegetable or chicken broth

1 tablespoon extra-virgin olive oil

1 pound extra-lean ground chicken

1 tablespoon curry powder

⅛ teaspoon cayenne pepper (optional)

sea salt and black pepper, to taste

1 tablespoon peeled and grated fresh ginger

1 cup diced fresh or frozen mango

1 carrot, finely grated

1 cup chopped baby kale

1 zucchini, grated

1 tablespoon tamari

1. Bring the quinoa and broth to a boil in a medium saucepan, reduce the heat to a simmer, cover, and cook for 10 to 12 minutes. Fluff the quinoa with a fork and set aside.

2. Heat the olive oil in a large skillet over medium heat, then add the ground chicken, curry powder, cayenne pepper, sea salt, and black pepper. Mix well and continue to stir until the chicken is thoroughly cooked, 7 to 10 minutes.

3. Once the chicken is cooked, add the quinoa, ginger, mango, carrot, kale, zucchini, and tamari. Lower the heat to a simmer and continue to stir for about 5 minutes, until the vegetables are cooked through.

4. Plate and serve!

No-fredo Spaghetti Squash with Chicken and Tomatoes

Who says going lower carb means that you have to give up spaghetti dinners and cheesy, creamy Alfredo sauce? Spaghetti squash gives you numerous options to still enjoy pasta-like meals. Personally, I feel pasta is really a vehicle for the sauce and toppings, so if you have a flavorful sauce such as this one, you won't miss the pasta and the spaghetti squash will be very satisfying.

Prep time: 15 minutes | *Cook time:* 45 minutes |
Makes: 4 servings

1 spaghetti squash, halved and deseeded

1½ teaspoons olive oil

3 cloves minced garlic, divided

2 cups water

1½ cups raw cashews

½ medium sweet onion, finely diced

2 cups unsweetened almond milk

¼ cup nutritional yeast

1 tablespoon lemon juice

2 large tomatoes, diced

2 cups baby spinach

8 ounces chicken breast, cooked, cubed

1 teaspoon red pepper flakes

sea salt and black pepper, to taste

1. Preheat the oven to 375°F and line a baking sheet with parchment paper.

2. Place the squash halves on the baking sheet with the flesh side up. Massage the flesh of the squash with the olive oil.

3. Spread 1 clove of minced garlic between the two squash halves, sprinkle with salt and pepper, and place on the baking sheet. Bake for 45 minutes.

4. While the squash is baking, bring 2 cups of water to a boil in a medium saucepan. Add the cashews, cover, turn off the heat, and soak for 5 minutes.

5. In a large skillet, heat the olive oil over medium-low heat. Sauté the onion and the remaining minced garlic and stir until the onion is translucent and the mixture is fragrant.

6. Drain the cashews and place them in a blender along with the onion and garlic mixture, unsweetened almond milk, nutritional yeast, lemon juice, and salt. Blend until smooth and creamy.

7. Remove the squash from the oven and let cool for 5 minutes. Using a gloved hand, hold each half up vertically and scrape out the flesh using a fork. Angel hair–like noodles should easily fall away from the skin.

8. In the same large skillet over very low heat, add the spaghetti squash and pour the cream sauce on top. Toss to combine, then add the tomatoes, spinach, and chicken and mix until the ingredients are heated through.

9. Plate in your favorite pasta bowls and add red pepper flakes, sea salt, and pepper to taste.

Healthy Avocado, Tuna, and Edamame Salad

This is my go-to lunch or quick dinner when my schedule gets hectic. You can make it the night before; just keep the dressing in a separate container until you're ready to eat. Good-quality canned tuna and organic edamame are staples to have on hand. The edamame provides great fiber and texture, and the extra protein will keep you satisfied. Some variations include using chicken, salmon, shrimp, beans, or lentils instead of the tuna. If you want to make a healthier "mayo," mash the avocado and mix it up with the vinegar, olive oil, and mustard.

Prep time: 15 to 20 minutes | *Cook time:* None | *Makes:* 2 servings

1½ teaspoons balsamic vinegar

1½ teaspoons Dijon mustard

1 tablespoon extra-virgin olive oil

sea salt and black pepper, to taste

1 (5- to 6-ounce) can or pouch tuna, drained and flaked

½ cup frozen edamame, thawed

¼ medium cucumber, diced (skin on or off—it will have more fiber with the peel left on)

1 celery stalk, diced

½ head endive, julienned

½ avocado, diced

2 cups chopped baby kale leaves

¼ cup alfalfa sprouts

2 tablespoons slivered almonds (or any nut/seed you prefer)

1. Combine the balsamic vinegar, mustard, olive oil, sea salt, and black pepper in a small bowl. Mix the dressing well, and set it aside.

2. Combine the remaining ingredients together in a large salad bowl.

3. Pour the desired amount of dressing over the salad, and toss well.

Hey Al, Where's My Fredo? Sauce

Alfredo sauce is one of my favorite comfort foods. We've already tried one version made with cashews. Here's a different take that shows just how versatile cauliflower can be. I've mentioned the benefit of going dairy-free for the first few weeks of your sugar detox. Being such a mildly flavored vegetable, cauliflower can make soups and sauces taste very creamy—without the added calories from dairy. You can also stream or sauté the ingredients here, but I like to roast my cauliflower to add a depth to the flavor. You won't be disappointed.

Prep time: 5 minutes | *Cook time:* 20 minutes | *Makes:* 6 servings

1 head cauliflower large, chopped into florets

2 shallots, chopped

1 tablespoon avocado oil

2 cloves garlic, minced

½ cup nutritional yeast

1 cup organic, unsweetened, full-fat coconut milk

3 tablespoons lemon juice

1 teaspoon sea salt

1. Preheat your oven to 375°F and line a baking sheet with parchment paper.

2. Add the cauliflower florets and shallots to the baking sheet and pour the oil over them. Toss with your hands or a spatula to coat evenly. Bake for 20 minutes or until the cauliflower is fork-tender.

3. Transfer the cauliflower to a blender and add the garlic, nutritional yeast, coconut milk, lemon juice, and sea salt, then blend on high until the mixture is smooth and creamy.

4. Serve over your favorite spiralized veggies, edamame pasta, grilled chicken, or shrimp or store in the fridge for 2 to 3 days.

Spicy Tempeh Salad

If you've never tried tempeh before, this is a great recipe to get your taste buds wet. If you're not a fan of heat, skip the sriracha sauce.

Prep: 15 minutes | *Cook time:* 20 minutes | *Makes:* 4 servings

2 tablespoons coconut aminos or tamari

1 tablespoon balsamic vinegar

1 teaspoon sriracha sauce

1 teaspoon chili powder

½ teaspoon smoked paprika

¼ teaspoon sea salt, divided

8 ounces tempeh, sliced into thin strips

3 tablespoons lemon juice

2 tablespoons water

2 tablespoons tahini

⅛ teaspoon garlic powder

4 cups finely chopped baby kale

4 cups baby spinach

½ cup sliced daikon radish

2 tablespoons pine nuts

1. Preheat the oven to 375°F and line a baking sheet with parchment paper.

2. In a large mixing bowl, combine the coconut aminos, vinegar, sriracha, chili powder, paprika, and half of the salt.

3. Add the tempeh, stir, and set aside for 10 to 15 minutes as the mixture marinates.

4. Lay the strips of tempeh out evenly (but not overlapping) on your baking sheet and bake for 10 minutes. Flip the strips over and bake for another 10 minutes. Remove the pan from the oven. When the strips are cool enough to handle, break them into bite-size pieces.

5. Add the lemon juice, water, tahini, garlic powder, and the remaining salt to a large mixing bowl with the kale, spinach, and radish, and toss well to evenly distribute the dressing.

6. Divide the salad into four bowls, add the tempeh pieces, garnish with the pine nuts, and serve.

I Heart Smoked Salmon

You don't need a bagel to top with smoked salmon. This recipe gives you the best of both worlds: smoked salmon and organic bacon on a bed of greens with a tangy dressing.

Prep time: 15 minutes | *Cook time:* None |
Makes: 2 servings

1 clove garlic, minced

¼ cup extra-virgin olive oil

1½ tablespoons lemon juice

1 tablespoon red wine vinegar

¼ teaspoon sea salt

1 cup spinach leaves

2 romaine hearts, roughly chopped

¼ cup sliced radishes

4 slices cooked organic bacon, crumbled

4 ounces smoked salmon

1 tablespoon chopped chives

1 avocado, sliced

1. To make the dressing: Add the garlic, olive oil, lemon juice, red wine vinegar, and sea salt to a small jar or shaker bottle and shake well to blend.

2. Add the spinach and romaine to a large mixing bowl. Toss in the radishes, bacon, smoked salmon, and chives.

3. Divide the salad between two serving bowls, pour the dressing on top, add the avocado slices, and serve.

"Cheesy" Chicken and Broccoli Bake

Chicken, broccoli, and cheese are household favorites, and this recipe never disappoints. Plus, there's nothing better than a one-pan meal!

Prep time: 15 minutes | *Cook time:* 40 to 45 minutes | *Makes:* 4 servings

1¼ cups unsweetened, organic, full-fat coconut milk

3 tablespoons nutritional yeast

1 tablespoon tapioca flour

½ teaspoon cumin

½ teaspoon onion powder

½ teaspoon garlic powder

¾ cup organic chicken broth

1 pound chicken breasts, sliced into tenders

¼ teaspoon sea salt and pepper

5 cups broccoli florets

1 shallot, thinly sliced

½ cup sliced mushrooms

1. Preheat the oven to 400°F.

2. In a medium saucepan over medium-low heat, add the coconut milk, nutritional yeast, tapioca flour, cumin, onion powder, and garlic powder. Stir well to combine.

3. Bring to a simmer and stir in the chicken broth. Remove from the heat.

4. Place the chicken on a large roasting pan and season with sea salt and pepper.

5. Top the chicken with the broccoli, shallot, and mushrooms. Pour the coconut milk sauce on top.

6. Place the roasting pan in the oven and bake for 40 to 45 minutes.

7. Plate and serve with cauliflower rice or quinoa, or over a bed of fresh spinach.

Detox Green Soup

Consider this a warm bowl of detoxing nutrients to support your body, all while tasting pretty darn good! I like drinking this from a mug with the fireplace going and a kitty on my lap. In the summer, serve chilled.

Prep time: 15 minutes | *Cook time:* 35 minutes | *Makes:* 4 servings

3 cups chopped asparagus

10 cloves garlic, chopped

½ yellow onion, chopped

½ head broccoli, sliced into florets

1 tablespoon extra-virgin olive oil

2½ cups organic vegetable broth

2 cups baby spinach

salt and pepper, to taste

1. Preheat the oven to 350°F and line a baking sheet or roasting pan with parchment paper.

2. Place all of the veggies, except the spinach, on the baking sheet and season with salt and pepper to taste. Drizzle the olive oil over the veggies and shake the pan to mix and spread the oil.

3. Place the pan in the oven and bake for 15 minutes. Stir the veggies and bake an additional 15 minutes, or until the veggies have caramelized.

4. While the veggies are finishing, place the vegetable broth in a medium saucepan and simmer. Add the spinach to the broth and cook until it wilts, about 2 to 3 minutes.

5. Once the veggies are roasted, place them in a blender along with the broth and spinach. Puree until smooth and creamy. Add extra broth to thin the soup to your preferred consistency.

6. Pour into bowls or a wide mug, grab a good book and a blanket, and savor the goodness of self-care!

Coconut Curry Turmeric Cauliflower

This simple and easy recipe serves up some potent anti-inflammatory and detox power while providing a warm, satisfying dish. Enjoy it alone or serve with your favorite protein.

Prep time: 10 to 15 minutes | *Cook time:* 15 to 20 minutes | *Makes:* 4 servings

2 cups plain, unsweetened, full-fat coconut milk

1 tablespoon turmeric

1 tablespoon curry powder

1 teaspoon sea salt

1 teaspoon black pepper

1 head cauliflower, chopped into florets

1. Add the coconut milk, turmeric, curry powder, salt, and pepper to a large skillet over medium heat. Mix well, reduce the heat to low, and cook until the sauce bubbles.

2. Add the cauliflower florets, reduce the heat, cover, and simmer for 15 to 20 minutes or until the cauliflower is fork-tender.

3. Ladle the mixture into serving bowls, add a pinch more of turmeric or paprika for color, and serve.

Pesto Portobello BLT

Show me the bacon! Yes, you can still have some bacon from time to time. Remember, quality matters. When cutting down on carbs and bread, look to veggies to take their place. If you don't like mushrooms, you can stuff a raw bell pepper or even use heartier lettuce leaves like romaine for a BLT wrap.

Prep time: 10 minutes | *Cook time:* 20 minutes | *Makes:* 4 servings

8 slices organic bacon

4 large portobello mushroom caps

sea salt and black pepper, to taste

1 clove garlic, minced

1 cup chopped fresh basil

¼ cup pine nuts

1 lemon, juiced

¼ cup extra-virgin olive oil

1 cup spring mix greens

1 avocado, peeled and sliced

1 tomato, sliced

1. Preheat the oven to 400°F.

2. While the oven is preheating, cook the bacon to your preferred level of crispiness in a large skillet over medium-high heat. Allow it to cool on a paper towel–lined plate.

3. Place the mushroom caps facedown on a baking sheet and brush each cap with a bit of olive oil. Season them with sea salt and black pepper.

4. Bake the mushrooms in the oven for 10 minutes and then remove them and set aside.

5. As the mushrooms cool slightly, place the garlic, basil, pine nuts, lemon juice, and extra-virgin olive oil in your blender or food processer and blend until creamy.

6. Place each mushroom on a dinner or salad plate with a handful of spring mix in the center of each cap.

7. Layer on the sliced avocado, tomato, and bacon.

8. Spoon the pesto sauce from the blender over the top of each mushroom cap.

Easy Peasy Detox Side Salad

If you're looking for a quick side or a snack that's cool and refreshing, this one will fit the bill. Plus, nothing says "detox" like cilantro and parsley! Toss in a can of tuna, salmon, diced chicken, tofu, or beans and you have a nice meal too!

Prep time: 10 minutes | *Cook time:* None |
Makes: 1 serving

½ cucumber, sliced

½ avocado

2 teaspoons sunflower seeds

1½ teaspoons lemon juice

1½ teaspoons extra-virgin olive oil

1 tablespoon chopped fresh parsley

1 tablespoon chopped cilantro

⅛ teaspoon sea salt

1. Combine all of the ingredients in a medium mixing bowl and toss well.

2. Transfer to the serving bowl of your choice and enjoy or place in the fridge to chill and enjoy later that day.

Basic Detox Green Salad

Making a healthy meal doesn't have to be labor intensive. This delicious and nutritious meal takes mere minutes but will keep you energized for hours.

Prep time: 10 minutes | *Cook time:* None |
Makes: 2 servings

2 tablespoons Dijon mustard

1 tablespoon apple cider vinegar

1 tablespoon extra-virgin olive oil

1 (5- to 6-ounce) can or pouch tuna or salmon, drained

2 stalks celery, diced

2 cups spring mix greens

1 cup chopped baby spinach

1 cup chopped baby kale

1 carrot, shredded

1 pear, cored and diced, with peel left on

¼ cup sliced almonds

sea salt and black pepper, to taste

1. Prepare your dressing in a small bowl by whisking together the Dijon mustard, apple cider vinegar, and olive oil.

2. In a large mixing bowl, combine all of the remaining ingredients.

3. Pour the dressing on top. Toss well.

4. Divide the dressed salad between two serving bowls, season with salt and pepper to taste, and enjoy.

DINNER

Harvest's Bounty Soup

If this doesn't taste like fall in a bowl, I don't what know what does. Hearty butternut squash and roasted pumpkin are two of my favorite veggies and can be so versatile once you get past cutting into them. If you have a hard time handling a knife, you may want to opt for buying pre-cubed butternut squash and pumpkin in your fresh produce section. Omit the crème fraîche or sour cream if you are avoiding dairy, or use a vegan substitute.

Prep time: 15 minutes | *Cook time:* 75 minutes |
Makes: 4 servings

2 cups butternut squash, cut in half lengthwise and deseeded

2 cup pumpkin, halved and deseeded

2 tablespoons extra-virgin olive oil

2 teaspoons cinnamon

½ teaspoon ground cloves

½ teaspoon ground nutmeg

2 tart apples, peeled, cored, and sliced

2 large shallots, diced

1 tablespoon fresh ginger, grated

4 cups organic vegetable broth

1 teaspoon sea salt

½ cup pine nuts, coarsely chopped

¼ cup crème fraîche or sour cream

1. Preheat the oven to 425°F.

2. Place the butternut squash and pumpkin on a large baking sheet with the flesh side up.

3. Massage 1 tablespoon of the oil onto the squash and pumpkin.

4. Sprinkle both veggies with the cinnamon and cloves and bake in the oven for 45 minutes or until the veggies are fork-tender. The cooking time will vary depending on the size of your squash and pumpkin.

5. Remove the baking sheet from the oven and let the veggies cool. Use a spoon to scoop out the flesh of the veggies and set it aside. Discard the skins.

6. Heat 1 tablespoon of olive oil in a large pot over medium heat. Add the apples, onion, nutmeg, and ginger, and sauté for about 5 minutes, or until the onions and apples become soft.

7. Add the vegetable broth, cooked veggies, and half of the sea salt. Reduce the heat to a simmer for 15 minutes.

8. While the soup is simmering, toast the pine nuts in a large frying pan or in your toaster oven until they are lightly browned. Then set them aside.

9. Using an immersion blender, puree the soup until it reaches a creamy, thick consistency. If you do not have an immersion blender (recommended), pour the soup into a stand blender and puree in smaller batches to prevent liquid from frothing over or excess steam building up.

10. Pour the soup into four bowls and top with a tablespoon each of the pine nuts and crème fraîche. Finish with a sprinkle of cinnamon.

Not Your Nana's Meatloaves

Meatloaf may be comfort food for some, but for others it incites visions of dried-out meat in a loaf pan, covered with ketchup. This yummy take on an old staple is infused with veggies and extra plant protein and fiber. You can customize it to your preference by choosing your favorite healthy grain.

Prep time: 15 minutes | *Cook time:* 45 minutes |
Makes: 6 servings (2 muffins per serving)

1½ teaspoons extra-virgin olive oil

½ yellow onion, finely chopped

1 clove garlic, minced

¾ cup cooked grain of your choice, such as quinoa, amaranth, or wild rice

¾ pound extra-lean ground turkey

¾ cup cooked lentils

1 tomato, diced

1 cup chopped escarole

1 small bell pepper, deseeded and chopped

¼ cup diced mushrooms

1 tablespoon tamari

1 tablespoon Dijon mustard

1 tablespoon nutritional yeast

1 teaspoon turmeric

1 egg

½ cup no-sugar-added tomato sauce

sea salt and black pepper, to taste

1. Preheat the oven to 350°F. Prepare a muffin tin with paper cups or lightly grease each well with olive oil.

2. In a small skillet, heat the olive oil over medium heat and sauté your onions for 5 minutes or until they become translucent. Add the garlic and sauté for an additional minute, until fragrant. Remove from the heat.

3. Place the cooked grain, garlic/onion mix, turkey, lentils, tomato, escarole, bell pepper, mushrooms, tamari, mustard, nutritional yeast, turmeric, and egg in a large mixing bowl and stir well to combine. Add salt and pepper to taste.

4. Scoop the mixture into your muffin tin. Add a spoonful of tomato sauce to the top of each cup.

6. Bake for 30 to 40 minutes, or until the turkey is fully cooked and the muffins are golden brown.

7. Remove from the oven and place 2 muffins on each serving plate. Serve with your favorite side salad and steamed or sautéed veggies.

Thanksgiving in a Bowl Bake

You don't have to wait until Thanksgiving to whip up this type of dish. This has the makings of comfort food in a bowl.

Prep time: 15 minutes | *Cook time:* 45 minutes | *Makes:* 4 servings

1 tablespoon extra-virgin olive oil

1 pound extra-lean ground turkey

1 yellow onion, finely chopped

2 cloves garlic, minced

1 teaspoon dried rosemary

1 teaspoon dried thyme

1 teaspoon sea salt

1 cup chopped kale leaves

1 cup halved Brussels sprouts

1 cup chopped beets

1 cup chopped carrot

2 stalks chopped celery

¾ cup unsweetened, organic, full-fat coconut milk

¼ cup chopped pecans

1 tablespoon no-sugar-added dried cranberries

1. Preheat the oven to 400°F.

2. Heat the oil in a large skillet over medium-high heat, then add the turkey to the pan, sautéing until fully cooked. Spoon the cooked turkey into a roasting pan.

3. Pour off any excess fat from the skillet. Return the skillet to the stovetop, add the onion and garlic, and cook for 3 to 5 minutes until the onion becomes translucent.

4. Mix in the dried herbs and sea salt. Add the kale, Brussels sprouts, beets, carrot, and celery to the skillet and sauté for another 5 minutes.

5. Stir in the coconut milk and mix well.

6. Pour the vegetable mixture over the cooked turkey. Cover with a lid or foil and bake for 20 to 25 minutes or until the beets are tender.

7. Serve in your favorite bowls, garnish with the pecans and cranberries, and enjoy.

Who Needs Takeout Fried Rice

It is bound to happen. There is going to be a time when you simply want to have some greasy takeout. Keeping a bag of wild-caught shrimp and organic cauliflower rice in the freezer at all times makes this a quick, easy-to-assemble meal. If you have fresh cauliflower, you can use that in place of frozen. Rather than make a not-so-healthy choice, give this recipe a try. Feel free to swap out the shrimp with another protein, such as tofu, chicken, or beef, to make whichever type of fried rice you are craving.

Prep time: 10 minutes | *Cook time:* 15 minutes |
Makes: 4 servings

2 teaspoons avocado oil, divided

1 pound shrimp, peeled and deveined

½ teaspoon chili powder

2 eggs

4 cups cauliflower rice, thawed

1 large carrot, diced

2 red or orange bell peppers, diced

1½ cups edamame, thawed and shelled

½ cup green peas

¼ cup coconut aminos or tamari

¼ cup cashews, chopped

4 scallions, sliced

1. Heat 1½ teaspoons of the oil in a large skillet over medium heat. Add the shrimp and chili powder and sauté for 3 minutes. Turn the shrimp and cook for another 3 minutes or until all of the shrimp is fully cooked. Transfer the shrimp to a medium bowl and set aside.

2. Using the same skillet, scramble and cook the eggs, then add them to the bowl with the shrimp.

3. Drizzle the skillet with the rest of the avocado oil and add the cauliflower rice, carrot, bell peppers, edamame, and peas, and sauté over medium heat. Using a spatula, pat the veggies down and let brown for 3 to 4 minutes, until they are a bit crispy. Stir, pat down again, and cook for 5 more minutes.

4. Pour in the coconut aminos and mix well.

5. Return the shrimp and egg back to the skillet and mix well. Divide between your serving bowls and garnish with the cashews and scallions.

Garlicky Chicken with Quinoa and Asparagus

A winning combination, zesty chicken and my favorite veggie—asparagus. You can also use legs and wings if you don't have thighs on hand. By the way, it you get the "asparagus pee," thank your genes for that! Cooking your quinoa in broth instead of plain water will help to infuse more flavor. You can even add some onion or garlic powder to the saucepan to add more zest.

Prep time: 10 minutes | *Cook time:* 20 minutes | *Makes:* 4 servings

¼ cup extra-virgin olive oil, plus more for grilling

6 cloves garlic, minced

2 tablespoons chili powder

2 teaspoons sea salt

1 teaspoon black pepper

2 pounds chicken thighs

1 large bunch of fresh asparagus, woody ends removed

1 cup quinoa

2 cups organic vegetable or chicken broth

1 tablespoon chopped parley

1. Combine the olive oil, minced garlic, chili powder, sea salt, and black pepper in a small bowl. Stir well.

2. Pour the mixture into a zip-top bag and add the chicken thighs. Shake well and place in the refrigerator to marinate while you work on the next steps.

3. Preheat your grill to medium heat or your oven to 400°F.

4. On a large plate, drizzle the asparagus with extra-virgin olive oil and season with sea salt and pepper. Set aside until you are ready to grill.

5. Add the quinoa and broth to a medium saucepan over high heat and bring to a boil.

6. Once boiling, reduce the heat to a simmer. Cover with a lid and simmer for 12 to 15 minutes or until all of the broth is absorbed. Remove the quinoa from the heat and fluff with a fork.

7. Place the chicken thighs on the grill and cook for 7 to 10 minutes per side or until cooked through. Or, place them on a large baking sheet and bake, turning them over after 15 minutes and baking for an additional 15 minutes.

8. Grill the asparagus for 6 to 7 minutes, until tender, or cook in the oven for 10 minutes.

9. Serve the chicken and asparagus over a scoop of quinoa. Season to taste. Garnish with a pinch of chopped parsley.

Pan-Seared Salmon with Almonds and Herbed Kohlrabi

If you have never tried kohlrabi, here's the perfect chance to! This veggie is great cooked or raw. Just be sure to remove the bitter, fibrous outer skin with a sharp knife. Using a green or purple kohlrabi will not only look pretty but also taste amazing and be a powerful source of detoxifying nutrients. When it is combined with the omega-3s in wild-caught salmon, you've got one nutrient-dense meal.

Prep time: 10 minutes | *Cook time:* 15 minutes | *Makes:* 2 servings

1 anchovy (optional but definitely worth keeping in)

½ cup finely chopped fresh parsley

2 cloves garlic, minced

1½ tablespoons lemon juice

¼ teaspoon sea salt

¼ cup extra-virgin olive oil, divided

10 ounces wild-caught salmon fillet

3 cups chopped kohlrabi

½ cup sliced almonds

1. Add the anchovy to a small mixing bowl and mash it with a fork.

2. Mix in the parsley, garlic, lemon, salt, and three-quarters of the oil. Set the herb sauce aside.

3. Place the remaining oil in a medium skillet and place the salmon skin-side down on the skillet while it is still cold. Turn the heat up to medium, cooking the fish for a total of 10 to 12 minutes depending on the thickness of the fillet and how rare you like your fish.

4. When the skin releases easily from the pan, flip the salmon over and cook for an additional minute. Remove from the pan and set aside.

5. In the same skillet, sauté the kohlrabi for 2 to 3 minutes, until lightly browned.

6. Divide the kohlrabi between two serving plates, add salmon to each, and top off with the herb sauce and sliced almonds.

Pecan-Crusted Halibut with Broccolini

A well-balanced anti-inflammatory and detox-supporting diet should include wild-caught fish a couple of times per week. Besides salmon, mahi mahi and rainbow trout are good options for this recipe. Plus, who doesn't love a one-pan meal?!

Prep time: 5 minutes | *Cook time:* 15 minutes | *Makes:* 2 servings

¼ cup very finely chopped pecans

1 scallion, very finely chopped

¼ teaspoon sea salt, plus more to taste

½ teaspoon Italian seasoning

½ teaspoon lemon juice

1 tablespoon extra-virgin olive oil, divided

8 ounces wild-caught halibut fillet, sliced into 4-ounce portions

1 large bunch broccolini

black pepper, to taste

1. Preheat the oven to 350°F. Line a baking sheet with parchment paper.

2. In a small bowl, combine the pecans, scallion, salt, Italian seasoning, lemon juice, and a third of the oil. Stir well.

3. Rub a third of the oil over both sides of the halibut fillets and place them in the baking sheet with the skin side down. Place the pecan dressing directly over the fish and gently pat it down to seal in the flavor.

4. Coat the broccolini with the remaining oil and season to taste with sea salt and pepper. Add the seasoned broccolini to the baking sheet next to the fish.

5. Place the baking sheet in the oven and bake for 12 to 15 minutes. When the halibut is fully cooked it will flake easily with a fork. Plate the fillets with the broccolini. Garnish with a bit more lemon juice and serve.

Cleansing Crucifers and Legume Soup

This soup is not just for cleansing and detox but is wonderful any time of the year. I like to use both red and green lentils to add color. Make this in large batches and freeze for a quick, nourishing meal on demand.

Prep time: 10 minutes | *Cook time:* 35 minutes | *Makes:* 6 servings

3 tablespoons extra-virgin olive oil

1 large yellow onion, diced

3 stalks celery, diced

2 medium carrots, diced

4 cloves garlic, minced

2 cups chopped broccoli florets

2 cups chopped cauliflower florets

4 cups chopped kale leaves

2 cups chopped bok choy

8 cups organic vegetable broth

2 cups lentils, cooked

1 cup cannellini beans, rinsed and drained

sea salt and black pepper, to taste

1. Heat a large stockpot over medium heat. Add the olive oil and heat it through.

2. Add the onion, celery, and carrots and sauté for 10 minutes, or until the onions are translucent.

3. Add the garlic and sauté for 3 minutes.

4. With the carrots, celery, and onion now softened, add the broccoli, cauliflower, kale, bok choy, and vegetable broth to the pot and bring the soup to a boil. Reduce the heat to low and let the soup simmer for 20 minutes.

5. Add the cooked lentils and beans to the soup and continue to simmer for another 3 to 5 minutes to allow the legumes to heat thoroughly.

6. Ladle the soup into your favorite bowls or mugs and season it to taste with sea salt and black pepper. Serve and lift a spoon to your health.

Under-Pressure Chicken Curry

One of the keys to eating healthier is to make sure that your food is also very flavorful. You have been used to eating things that taste sweet, so now I will be challenging you to broaden your flavor palette as we take a culinary tour around the world. This recipe requires a pressure cooker. If you do not have one, add it to your holiday, birthday, or anniversary wish list pronto! You'll thank me later! In the meantime, you can use a slow cooker on the low setting for 6 to 8 hours. Feel free to serve this with brown rice, cauliflower rice, or quinoa.

Prep time: 10 minutes | *Cook time:* 30 minutes | *Makes:* 4 servings

1 tablespoon extra-virgin olive oil

1 yellow onion, chopped

3 cloves garlic, minced

1 tablespoon minced or grated fresh ginger

1 tablespoon curry powder

1½ teaspoons cumin

1 teaspoon Chinese five-spice powder

½ teaspoon sea salt

1½ cups organic chicken or vegetable broth

1 pound chicken breast

1 cup unsweetened, full-fat organic coconut milk

1 tablespoon chopped cilantro

1 tablespoon lime juice

1. Turn your pressure cooker to sauté mode and heat the oil. Once the pot is heated, sauté the onion for 3 to 4 minutes, then add the garlic, ginger, curry powder, Chinese five-spice powder, cumin, and salt, and continue to cook for 1 more minute.

2. Add the broth to the pot, stirring and scraping the bottom to combine and free those lovely brown bits of flavor from the bottom of the pot. Next, add in the chicken breast and close the lid.

3. Turn and seal your pressure cooker to manual/pressure cooking mode and set to cook for 5 minutes at high pressure. Remember, it'll take a few minutes for the cooker to come up to pressure. Once the 5 minutes of high-pressure cooking are completed, do a quick manual pressure release. Remove the cooked chicken to a plate and set aside.

4. Turn the pressure cooker back to sauté mode and pour in the coconut milk. Stir the liquid frequently as it reduces by half, 12 to 15 minutes. When the sauce is thick and creamy, add the cilantro and lime juice. Stir once more and turn off the pressure cooker.

5. Plate your chicken and cover liberally with your curry sauce.

Roll Your Own Sushi

Most of my friends know that sushi is one of my favorite foods, but not when it's loaded down with sugary sauces or dipped in batter and fried. Here's a chance to make some healthy sushi rolls at home that will capitalize on detoxifying nutrients such as vitamins A, B6, and C, fiber, and iodine. Try to opt for lower-mercury fish.

Prep time: 15 minutes | *Cook time:* 5 minutes |
Makes: 2 servings

½ tablespoon olive oil

3 cups cauliflower rice

2 tablespoons rice vinegar

2 teaspoons tapioca starch

4 large nori sheets, cut in half

1 small avocado, sliced

½ medium cucumber, sliced into thin strips

½ red bell pepper, sliced into thin strips

6 ounces of any of the following: smoked salmon, sushi-grade salmon, sushi-grade tuna, grilled chicken or fish, or tofu

2 tablespoons tamari or coconut aminos, to serve

1 teaspoon wasabi, to serve

pickled ginger slices (optional), to serve

1. In a large skillet, heat the olive oil over medium heat and sauté the cauliflower rice for 3 minutes. Add the rice vinegar and stir, cooking the rice for 2 more minutes.

2. Add the tapioca starch, mix well, and remove from heat.

3. Pour the rice mixture into a wire mesh strainer to drain excess liquid and pat it down with a paper towel. Let it continue to drain in the strainer while you move on to the next step.

4. Place the nori sheets on a bamboo sushi roll mat if you have one. If not, any flat surface will do. Scoop the cauliflower rice onto the nori with a spoon, pressing down and spreading the rice in a thin layer on the sheets. Leave the top inch of each sheet uncovered.

5. Starting with the end of the nori closest to you, add your preferred combo of avocado, cucumber, pepper, and the protein of your choice, placing them about an inch from the bottom and layering them in a line that is parallel to the bottom of the nori sheet.

6. For a traditional roll, start at the end closest to you and begin to roll the nori upward. With a sharp knife, slice each roll into 6 to 8 pieces. Plate and serve with the tamari, wasabi, and pickled ginger, if using.

Tip: For a less precise roll, opt for a hand roll. Add the rice the same way but place the ingredients for the middle of the roll on a diagonal, and roll up like a cornucopia. Plate and serve with the tamari, wasabi, and pickled ginger.

Chicken Shawarma

I have to make a confession. Every time I see or hear the word "shawarma" I immediately think of the Marvel Universe. Therefore, I hope this salad bowl full of detox-supporting nutrients and spices powers you up like Tony Stark or some other superhero! If you want to be more plant forward with this recipe, swap out the beans, lentils, or chickpeas for the chicken.

Prep time: 10 minutes | *Cook time:* 20 minutes |
Makes: 4 servings

1 pound chicken breasts, sliced into thin strips

½ teaspoon sea salt

½ teaspoon black pepper, plus more to taste

½ teaspoon ground cinnamon, plus more to taste

½ teaspoon turmeric

½ teaspoon garlic powder

½ teaspoon onion powder

1 teaspoon paprika

1 tablespoon cumin

2 tablespoons extra-virgin olive oil

¼ cup tahini

2 tablespoons water

juice of ½ lemon

4 cups spring mix greens

2 tomatoes, diced

1 cucumber, diced

cayenne pepper, to taste

1. In a large mixing bowl, combine the chicken, salt, pepper, cinnamon, turmeric, garlic powder, onion powder, paprika, cumin, and olive oil. With clean hands, massage the mixture well and be sure to coat each strip of chicken with the spices.

2. Place a large skillet on the stove over medium heat and pour the chicken mixture into the skillet. Cook the chicken for 8 to 10 minutes, or until it is thoroughly cooked.

3. While the chicken is cooking, prepare the dressing in a small bowl by combining the tahini, water, and lemon juice. Whisk well and set aside.

4. Toss the spring mix with the tomatoes and cucumber. When the chicken is done, add it to the salad and top with the tahini dressing. Toss all ingredients to mix well.

5. Divide the salad between four serving bowls. Add salt, pepper, and a pinch of cayenne pepper to taste, and serve.

Shish Kebobs with Citrus Avocado Sauce

A basic kebob recipe can become a staple that affords you the versatility to make any number of delicious combination throughout the year. Swap out the protein source with lamb, chicken, or beef. If you want to convert this to a meatless meal, use tofu or make veggie kebobs. Cook the kebobs in the oven or throw them on the grill if you can.

Prep time: 10 minutes | *Cook time:* 10 minutes | *Makes:* 5 servings

1 pound wild-caught shrimp, peeled and deveined

1 large onion, sliced into wedges

8 ounces baby portobello mushrooms

2 bell peppers, sliced into 1-inch pieces

1 bulb fennel, sliced into 1-inch pieces

1 small green or yellow zucchini, sliced into 1-inch pieces

1 teaspoon onion powder

1 teaspoon garlic powder

4 tablespoons extra-virgin olive oil, divided

10 metal or wooden skewers

1½ teaspoons sea salt, divided

juice of ½ lemon

juice of ½ lime

1 avocado, peeled, pitted, and roughly chopped

1. Preheat the oven to 400°F. Line a baking sheet with aluminum foil.

2. In a large mixing bowl, combine the shrimp, onion, mushrooms, peppers, fennel, zucchini, onion powder, garlic powder, and half of the oil and mix well to coat and distribute the seasonings.

3. Thread the seasoned shrimp and veggies onto the skewers, alternating between them and spreading the ingredients equally along the skewers. Spread the skewers across the baking sheet.

4. Sprinkle a pinch of salt over the threaded kebobs and place the sheet in the oven. Roast for 5 minutes, turn the kebobs over, and cook for 5 minutes more or until the shrimp is fully cooked through.

5. With the kebobs in the oven, it's time to make the dressing. Place the remaining oil, remaining salt, lemon juice, lime juice, and avocado in your food processor or blender. Blend until creamy. If the dressing is too thick, add a teaspoon of water at a time until it thins to your desired consistency.

6. Remove the kebobs from the oven and plate. Drizzle the citrus avocado dressing over each kebob and enjoy.

Asia-Inspired Nutty Chicken Salad

This recipe combines some of my favorites: chicken, peanuts, and broccoli. I love Asian flavors, and I hope you enjoy a good culinary world tour too.

Prep time: 25 minutes | *Cook time:* 10 minutes |
Makes: 4 servings

2 tablespoons coconut oil, divided

1¼ pounds chicken breast, diced

½ cup water chestnuts, drained

⅓ cup all-natural, no-added-sugar peanut butter (almond or cashew butter also work well, but you may need a bit more oil to thin out the dressing)

1 tablespoon tamari

juice of 1 lime

1 tablespoon peeled and grated ginger

1 clove garlic, minced

1 teaspoon Chinese five-spice powder

¼ cup water

1 head broccoli (stalk and florets), chopped

1 red bell pepper, chopped

1 carrot, chopped

⅓ cup raw chopped peanuts, to serve

sea salt and black pepper, to taste

3 scallions, chopped, to serve

1. Add 1 tablespoon of coconut oil to a large skillet or wok over medium heat. Add the chicken and sauté for 5 minutes.

2. Toss in the water chestnuts and continue to cook for 5 more minutes, or until the chicken is completely cooked.

3. Add the peanut butter, tamari, lime juice, remaining coconut oil, ginger, garlic, Chinese five-spice powder, and water to a blender or food processor and blend until smooth. Set aside.

4. Combine the veggies in a large serving bowl. Top the veggies with the cooked chicken and water chestnuts, and stir.

Pour on the dressing and toss well. Garnish with the chopped peanuts and scallions.

5. Season with sea salt and black pepper to taste and serve.

My Favorite Mahi Pepita Pesto

I know many people are always looking for ways to incorporate more fish dishes into their dinner rotations. This one is not only quick and easy, but brings a lot of flavor to the party too. Any milder white-fleshed fish will work well. I do not recommend consuming tilapia though, as finding wild-caught tilapia is nearly impossible. The majority of tilapia is farm-raised, exposing you to antibiotics, pesticides, and various other chemicals. Furthermore, tilapia has more omega-6s than omega-3s.

Prep time: 15 minutes | *Cook time:* 6 to 8 minutes | *Makes:* 4 servings

1 cup packed fresh parsley

¼ cup packed fresh dill

½ cup chopped pepitas

2 teaspoons coconut oil

1 scallion, chopped

juice of 1 lemon

2 cloves garlic, minced

2 teaspoons olive oil

20 ounces wild-caught mahi mahi fillets

4 cups baby spinach

4 cups arugula

sea salt and black pepper, to taste

1 lemon, sliced in wedges

1. Create your pesto by blending the parsley, dill, chopped pepitas, coconut oil, scallion, lemon juice, and garlic in a blender or food processor until a thick paste forms. You can thin it to your desired consistency by adding more oil or lemon juice.

2. Heat the olive oil in a large skillet over medium-high heat. Season both sides of your fish with salt and pepper and place it in the pan.

3. Fry the fish for 3 to 4 minutes per side, depending on the thickness of your fillets. The fish should be solid white to slightly golden brown and easily flake with a fork when finished.

4. Prepare four serving plates by placing ½ cup of spinach and ½ cup of arugula on each plate, creating a bed of greens for the fish. Place your cooked mahi mahi on the greens and spoon the pesto sauce on top. Season with sea salt and black pepper to taste, and serve with lemon wedges.

Savory Meatballs with Oven-Roasted Veggies

This is a perfect recipe to help support your organs of detoxification with cruciferous vegetables. Balsamic vinegar adds caramelization and intense flavor to the veggies, so be sure to choose a top-quality balsamic. As for the proteins, invest in good-quality, organic, grass-fed beef, pork, chicken, or turkey.

Prep time: 15 minutes | *Cook time:* 30 minutes | *Makes:* 4 servings

1 pound meat of choice

1 teaspoon chopped fresh thyme

1 teaspoon chopped fresh parsley

1 teaspoon chopped fresh rosemary

2 cloves garlic, minced

½ teaspoon sea salt, divided

3 cups Brussels sprouts, trimmed and halved

3 cups cauliflower florets

1 tablespoon balsamic vinegar

2 teaspoons avocado oil

1. Preheat the oven to 400°F and line a baking sheet with parchment paper.

2. In a medium mixing bowl, combine the meat, thyme, parsley, rosemary, garlic, and half of the sea salt. Dive in with clean hands to mix the ingredients well. Roll a tablespoon of the meat mixture into a ball and place it on the parchment-lined baking sheet. Repeat with the remaining meat mixture.

3. After all the meat is rolled into balls, add the Brussels sprouts and cauliflower to a large bowl with the vinegar, avocado oil, and remaining sea salt. Stir well to fully coat with the oil and vinegar.

4. Pour the veggies onto the baking sheet next to the meatballs, and bake for 30 minutes.

Grilled Shrimp Spinach Slaw Salad

This salad provides a pleasing balance between the hot shrimp and the cool salad fixings; plus, the liquids used to sauté the shrimp make a tasty dressing.

Prep time: 20 minutes | *Cook time:* 4 to 6 minutes | *Makes:* 4 servings

½ cup packed chopped fresh parsley

juice of 3 limes

¼ cup extra-virgin olive oil

1 teaspoon onion powder

1 teaspoon garlic powder

2 pounds raw shrimp, peeled and deveined

1 cup shredded green or purple cabbage

1 cup shredded jicama

1 cup shredded broccoli stalks

1 cup baby spinach

1 cup halved cherry tomatoes

1 carrot, shredded

1 avocado, peeled and diced

nutritional yeast, sea salt, and black pepper, to taste

1. To make the dressing: In your food processor or blender combine the parsley, lemon juice, onion powder, garlic powder, and olive oil. Blend well until smooth.

2. Heat your skillet over medium-high heat. Add the shrimp and three-quarters of the dressing.

3. Sauté the shrimp for 2 to 3 minutes per side until thoroughly cooked.

4. In a large serving bowl combine the remaining vegetable ingredients. When the shrimp is fully cooked, pour the entire contents of your skillet over the top of the salad bowl. Season with sea salt and pepper to taste, toss well, and serve.

Steakhouse Strip Salad

I love a great steak salad made with local, grass-fed, organic beef. Feel free to swap out the greens in this recipe for other greens of your choice, but bear in mind, with detox as our goal, kale provides just what your detox organs are calling for. Chicken, fish, and shrimp also work well with this base salad. If you want a more plant-forward meal, ditch the steak and opt for sautéed tofu or a variety of your favorite beans.

Prep time: 10 minutes | *Cook time:* 35 minutes | *Makes:* 4 servings

1 red bell pepper, deseeded and sliced into strips

1 orange bell pepper, deseeded and sliced into strips

¼ teaspoon sea salt

⅓ cup extra-virgin olive oil, divided

½ cup red onion, finely sliced

1 cucumber, diced

4 cups finely chopped kale leaves

1 cup halved cherry tomatoes

¾ cup diced pitted kalamata olives

3 tablespoons balsamic or red wine vinegar

½ teaspoon oregano

juice of 1 lemon

1 clove garlic, minced

⅛ teaspoon black pepper

12 ounces organic, grass-fed beef tenderloin

½ cup nutritional yeast

1. Preheat the oven to 425°F. Line a baking sheet with parchment paper.

2. In a large mixing bowl, combine the peppers, salt, and ½ tablespoon of the olive oil. Mix well to completely coat the peppers. Place the peppers on the baking sheet and roast in the oven for 20 minutes.

3. While the peppers are roasting, combine the remaining vegetables in a large salad bowl and set aside.

4. Prepare the dressing by mixing the remaining olive oil, vinegar, oregano, lemon juice, minced garlic, remaining sea salt, and pepper together in a small bowl. Stir well and set aside.

5. When the peppers are roasted, remove them from the oven and allow them to cool for a few minutes, then add them to the salad bowl with the other veggies.

6. Add just enough oil to coat the bottom of a large cast-iron skillet, and heat on the stovetop over medium heat. Place your steak in the skillet and cook for 4 to 5 minutes per side, depending on the size and thickness of your steak. Cook medium rare to medium.

7. Remove the steak from the skillet and let it rest for 5 minutes before cutting it into thin strips.

8. Pour the dressing over the salad and toss well to distribute. Plate the salad and add strips of steak and nutritional yeast over the top, toss, and serve.

Garlic Lemon Shrimp and Veggies

Eating healthy and low sugar doesn't mean you have to sacrifice flavor or easy meal prep. This recipe only requires one sheet pan, which means quick, easy cleanup.

Prep time: 15 minutes | *Cook time:* 15 minutes |
Makes: 2 servings

2 cups asparagus, woody ends trimmed

1 cup broccoli florets

1 cup halved Brussel sprouts

12 ounces raw shrimp, deveined, tails off

3 tablespoons extra-virgin olive oil

2 cloves garlic, minced

1 lemon, sliced

⅛ teaspoon sea salt, plus more to taste

1. Preheat your oven to 400°F. Line a baking sheet with parchment paper.

2. In a large mixing bowl, combine the asparagus, broccoli, Brussels sprouts, shrimp, oil, and garlic. Mix well to combine.

3. Pour the contents of the bowl onto the baking sheet and give it a shake to evenly spread the ingredients out. Use a spatula to scrap the bowl, getting all of the oil and garlic onto the pan.

4. Add the lemon slices and salt.

5. Pop the pan in the oven and bake for 15 minutes, turning the contents over halfway through the baking time. When the shrimp are fully cooked they will turn a bright orange-pink.

6. Remove the pan from the oven, plate, season with sea salt and black pepper to taste, and serve.

Veggie Medley Stir Fry with Zingy Chicken

I love to make stir-fry whenever I need to use up some veggies in the fridge or we need to hit our veggies intake goals for the day. No need for rice, but if you really want an extra veggie serving, place the stir-fry on a bed of cauliflower or kohlrabi rice.

Prep time: 10 minutes | *Cook time:* 20 minutes |
Makes: 4 servings

⅓ cup tamari or coconut aminos

2 cloves garlic, minced

1 tablespoon peeled and grated fresh ginger

1 tablespoon coconut oil

20 ounces chicken breast, sliced into cubes

2 shallots, diced

2 stalks celery, sliced

1 red bell pepper, diced

1 carrot, shredded

¾ cup snap peas

½ cup sliced mushrooms

2 cups chopped broccoli florets

2 cups chopped kale leaves

sesame seeds, for garnish

1. Prepare your sauce in a small mixing bowl by combining the tamari, garlic, and ginger. Stir well and set aside.

2. Heat the coconut oil in a large skillet or wok over medium heat. Add the chicken and shallots and sauté for 10 minutes.

3. Toss in all the remaining veggies except for the kale. Sauté for another 5 minutes.

4. Pour the sauce into the pan and stir well to mix. Place the kale on top and stir again. Continue to cook for 1 to 2 minutes to heat the kale. Once it has begun to wilt, remove the pan from the heat.

5. Place into bowls, garnish with sesame seeds, and serve.

DESSERT

Where's the Drive-In? Chocolate Milkshake

Grab a couple old-time milkshake glasses and two paper or metal straws and enjoy this guilt-free chocolate shake. If you're craving a frozen treat, pour into popsicle molds or ice-cube trays and freeze for a fudgy frozen dessert.

Prep time: 10 minutes | *Cook time:* None |
Makes: 2 serving

1 avocado, chopped

2 cups unsweetened almond milk

2 tablespoons nut or seed butter

2 scoops chocolate protein powder

½ tablespoon unsweetened cocoa powder

1½ teaspoons ground cinnamon

½ teaspoon ground nutmeg

¼ teaspoon vanilla extract

2 cups baby greens, spinach, or kale

1 teaspoon chia seeds (for garnish)

1. Add all of the ingredients except the chia seeds into your blender or food processer and blend until smooth and creamy.

2. Pour into your tall milkshake glasses, sprinkle on the chia seeds, add a pinch more spices to top, and serve.

3. For a creamy frozen dessert, pour into molds and freeze for at least 3 hours.

Chocolate Pumpkin Spice Chia Pudding

Pureed pumpkin is a useful staple in a lower-carbohydrate, sugar-free lifestyle. Packed full of flavor and nutrients, it provides the texture and consistency for comfort foods and desserts. It's combined with chia seeds, which I like to call "nature's Pop Rocks." I guarantee you won't miss the sugar in this satisfying dessert pudding.

Prep time: 5 minutes, plus 30 minutes to overnight to chill | *Cook time:* None | *Makes:* 2 servings

¼ cup chia seeds

¾ cup unsweetened almond milk

1 tablespoon unsweetened cocoa powder, plus more to taste

¼ cup pureed pumpkin

¼ teaspoon ground cinnamon

⅛ teaspoon ground nutmeg

⅛ teaspoon cloves

2 tablespoons unsweetened coconut or almond yogurt, divided

1. In a large mixing bowl, combine all of the ingredients except the yogurt. Mix well, ensuring that all of the chia seeds are evenly spread. Refrigerate 30 minutes to overnight to thicken and allow the flavors to marry.

2. Once thoroughly chilled, scoop the pudding into your favorite dessert bowl and place a dollop of the coconut or almond yogurt on top. Add a pinch of additional spices, if desired, and serve.

Macadamia Mania

Craving a bit of tropical island flair? This dessert whips up quickly but satisfies. Macadamia nuts are high in fat, which will keep you full and help to balance the carbohydrate from the berries.

Prep time: 5 minutes, plus 30 minutes to soak |
Cook time: None | *Makes:* 6 servings

1½ cups macadamia nuts, soaked for at least 30 minutes

1 tablespoon coconut oil, melted

¼ teaspoon ground cinnamon

¼ teaspoon unsweetened cocoa powder

¼ teaspoon vanilla extract

1 cup fresh strawberries

1 cup fresh blackberries

1. Add the macadamia nuts, coconut oil, cinnamon, cocoa powder, and vanilla extract to a food processor or high-speed blender and blend to a smooth, creamy consistency. If needed, add a teaspoon of water at a time to thin the mixture to your desired consistency.

2. Place the nut dip in the center of a serving dish with the berries arranged around the dip. Sprinkle a little cinnamon or cocoa powder on the berries, if desired.

3. Grab a few toothpicks or seafood forks, skewer a berry, and begin dipping!

Nuts over Chocolate

If cravings are really getting the best of you, I suggest you give this recipe a try before caving in. Remember our chat about the use of nonnutritive sweeteners? In the face of casting all your hard work aside, ¼ teaspoon of monk fruit sweetener is definitely the lesser of two evils. If you need a snack pronto, forgo warming them in the oven and just mix all the ingredients and enjoy.

Prep time: 2 minutes | *Cook time:* 5 to 7 minutes | *Makes:* 2 servings

½ cup almonds, pecans, or walnuts

1 tablespoon melted coconut oil

1 teaspoon unsweetened cocoa powder

¼ teaspoon sea salt

¼ teaspoon ground cinnamon

¼ teaspoon ground nutmeg

½ teaspoon monk fruit sweetener

⅛ teaspoon vanilla extract

1. Preheat the oven or toaster oven to 375°F. Line a baking sheet with parchment paper.

2. In a medium bowl, combine all of the ingredients and mix well.

3. Pour the mixture onto the baking sheet and bake for 5 to 7 minutes.

4. Remove from the oven and enjoy!

Not Your Average Nut Butter Cups

Yup—we're not sorry either about this yummy and healthy snack. You can make these using paper baking cups or silicone molds. I just use my silicone muffin tray.

Prep time: 15 minutes, plus 60 minutes to chill | *Cook time:* None | *Makes:* 6 servings

¼ cup almond butter (or nut or seed butter of your choice)

2 tablespoons melted coconut oil, divided

1½ teaspoons vanilla extract

1½ teaspoons ground cinnamon

¼ teaspoon ground nutmeg

2 teaspoons unsweetened cocoa powder

¹⁄₁₆ teaspoon sea salt

¼ cup coconut butter

1. In a medium mixing bowl, stir the almond butter and half of the melted coconut oil together until smooth.

2. Add in the vanilla, cinnamon, nutmeg, cocoa, and salt. Stir well. Do not get nervous if the mixture stiffens up a bit as you add the ingredients to the almond butter and oil.

3. In another small mixing bowl, mix the remaining melted coconut oil and coconut butter together and stir until loose.

4. Fold the loose mixture from the small bowl into the stiffer mixture in the medium bowl until well combined.

5. Spoon the mixture into paper baking cups arranged on a small baking sheet or into silicone molds. Freeze for at least one hour or until the cups are completely hardened. Enjoy one at a time or keep them in the freezer until needed.

Frozen Fruit Nice Cream

This recipe also works great with pear, plum, nectarine, or even berries. As we have a few varieties of berries on our property and our freezer is always well stocked with our berry bounty, this is a welcome treat not only during the summer berry season but also over the winter.

Prep time: 5 minutes, plus 1 to 3 hours to freeze |
Cook time: None | *Makes:* 3 servings

1 cup frozen fruit

½ cup macadamia nut butter

¼ teaspoon ground cinnamon

¼ teaspoon vanilla extract

1. Add your chosen frozen fruit, nut butter, cinnamon, and vanilla to your food processor and blend until smooth. You may need to pause from time to time to scrape down the sides. Continue to blend to your desired consistency—you may prefer a chunkier ice cream versus a soft serve.

2. When it has reached your desired consistency, scoop the ice cream into serving bowls for immediate enjoyment. If you prefer a harder ice cream, scoop it into a freezer-safe container and freeze for 1 to 3 hours before digging in.

ADDENDUM

As this book was going to press the USDA released the updated 2020–2025 Dietary Guidelines for Americans. There are not too many differences, but we've gone from five guidelines to the following four:

1. Follow a healthy dietary pattern at every life stage.

2. Customize and enjoy nutrient-dense food and beverage choices to reflect personal preferences, cultural traditions, and budgetary considerations.

3. Focus on meeting food group needs with nutrient-dense foods and beverages, and stay within calorie limits.

4. Limit foods and beverages higher in added sugars, saturated fat, and sodium, and limit alcoholic beverages.

I do want to point out a few notable items for these new guidelines. The USDA opted to keep the current limits on added sugars, fat, sodium, and alcohol for adults unchanged despite the scientific committee's two recommendations to cut the limit on added sugars to 6 percent from 10 percent of daily calories and to reduce the alcohol limit for men to one drink per day. Unfortunately, the body of scientific evidence available in relation to diet-related diseases was not enough to update the guidelines. It is not surprising that food industry lobbyists and groups such as the American Beverage Association were present at public meetings in August 2020 to press their interests in keeping the limits on sugar and alcohol at the status quo.

On a positive note, some of the scientific committee's suggestions were followed. We finally see guidance offered for the pediatric population. Regarding sugar, it is suggested to limit added sugars to less than 10 percent of calories per day starting at age two. For kids under two years old, it is recommended to avoid foods and beverages with added sugars. The recommendation to limit saturated fat to less than 10 percent of daily calories also begins at age two. The limit for sodium remains at less than 2,300 milligrams per day; however the direction for children under 14 is to aim for even less than that.

At the end of the day, remember these are guidelines not gospel, and our earlier discussion on the overall dietary guidelines still promote your personal introspection as you progress through the remainder of this book.

If you feel so inclined to read the full report, please visit https://www.dietaryguidelines.gov/sites/default/files/2020 -12/Dietary_Guidelines_for_Americans_2020-2025.pdf.

BIBLIOGRAPHY

Anton, Stephen D., Azumi Hida, Kacey Heekin, et al. "Effects of Popular Diets without Specific Calorie Targets on Weight Loss Outcomes: Systematic Review of Findings from Clinical Trials." *Nutrients* 9, no. 8 (July 2017). https://pubmed.ncbi.nlm.nih.gov/28758964.

Basaranoglu, Metin, Gokcen Basaranoglu, Tevfik Sabuncu, and Hakan Senturk. "Fructose as a Key Player in the Development of Fatty Liver Disease." *World Journal of Gastroenterology* 19, no. 8 (2013): 1166–72. https://pubmed.ncbi.nlm.nih.gov/23482247.

Binder, Henry J., and Charles M. Mansbach II. "Nutrient Digestion and Absorption." In *Medical Physiology*. Amsterdam: Elsevier, 2016.

Centers for Disease Control and Prevention. "Adult Obesity Prevalence Maps." Accessed September 11, 2020. https://www.cdc.gov/obesity/data/prevalence-maps.html.

Centers for Disease Control and Prevention, Division of Diabetes Translation. "Diagnosed Diabetes." US Diabetes Surveillance System. Accessed September 11, 2020. https://gis.cdc.gov/grasp/diabetes/DiabetesAtlas.html.

DiNicolantonio, James J., and Amy Berger. "Added Sugars Drive Nutrient and Energy Deficit in Obesity: A New Paradigm." *Open Heart* 3, no. 2 (2016). https://doi.org/10.1136/openhrt-2016-000469.

Gaby, Alan. *Nutritional Medicine.* Concord, NH: Fritz Perlberg Publishing, 2017.

Genetic Science Learning Center. "Making SNPs Make Sense." Learn.Genetics. February 1, 2016. Accessed November 23, 2020.

Goss, Amy M., Barbara Gower, Taraneh Soleyamani, et al. "Effects of Weight Loss during a Very Low Carbohydrate Diet on Specific Adipose Tissue Depots and Insulin Sensitivity in Older Adults with Obesity: A Randomized Clinical Trial." *Nutrition & Metabolism* 17, no. 64 (2020). https://doi.org/10.1186/s12986-020-00481-9.

Havel, Peter J. "Dietary Fructose: Implications for Dysregulation of Energy Homeostasis and Lipid/Carbohydrate Metabolism." *Nutrition Reviews* 63, no. 5 (May 2005): 133–57. https://pubmed.ncbi.nlm.nih.gov/15971409.

Hodges, Romilly E., and Deanna M. Minich. "Modulation of Metabolic Detoxification Pathways Using Foods and Food-Derived Components: A Scientific Review with Clinical Application." *Journal of Nutrition and Metabolism* 2015 (June 2015). https://pubmed.ncbi.nlm.nih.gov/26167297.

Hyman, Mark. "Systems Biology, Toxins, Obesity, and Functional Medicine." *Alternative Therapies in Health and Medicine* 13, no. 2 (April 2007): S134–39. https://pubmed.ncbi.nlm.nih.gov/17405691.

Johnson, Rachel K., Lawrence J. Appel, Michael Brands, Barbara V. Howard, et al. "Dietary Sugars Intake and Cardiovascular Health: A Scientific Statement from the American Heart Association." *Circulation* 120, no. 11 (September 2009): 1011–20. https://pubmed.ncbi.nlm.nih.gov/19704096.

Jones, David S. *Textbook of Functional Medicine.* Gig Harbor, WA: Institute for Functional Medicine, 2010.

Kearns, Cristin E., Laura A. Schmidt, and Stanton A. Glantz. "Sugar Industry and Coronary Heart Disease Research: A Historical Analysis of Internal Industry Documents." *JAMA Internal Medicine* 176, no. 11 (November 2016): 1680–85. https://pubmed.ncbi.nlm.nih.gov/27 617709.

Kim, Ju Ah, Jin Young Kim, and Seung Wan Kang. "Effects of Dietary Detoxification Program on Serum Y-Glutamyltransferase, Anthropometric Data and Metabolic Biomarkers in Adults." *Journal of Lifestyle Medicine* 6, no. 2 (September 2016): 49–57. https://www.ncbi.nlm.nih.gov/pmc/articles/PMC5115202.

Klein, A. V., and H. Kiat. "Detox Diets for Toxin Elimination and Weight Management: A Critical Review of the Evidence." *Journal of Human Nutrition and Dietetics: The Official Journal of the British Dietetic Association* 28, no. 6 (December 2015): 675–86. https://pubmed.ncbi.nlm.nih.gov/25522674.

Liska, DeAnn, Michael Lyon, and David S. Jones. "Detoxification and Biotransformational Imbalances." *Explore* 2, no. 2 (2006): 122–40. https://pubmed.ncbi.nlm.nih.gov/16781626.

Mahan, Kathleen, and Janice L. Raymond. *Krause's Food & the Nutrition Care Process*. Philadelphia: Saunders, 2012.

Marchesini, Giulio, Elisabetta Bugianesi, Gabriele Forlani, et al. "Nonalcoholic Fatty Liver, Steatohepatitis, and the Metabolic Syndrome." *Hepatology* 37, no. 4 (April 2003): 917–23. https://pubmed.ncbi.nlm.nih.gov/12668987.

Myles, Ian A. "Fast Food Fever: Reviewing the Impacts of the Western Diet on Immunity." *Nutrition Journal* 13, no. 1 (June 2014). https://nutritionj.biomedcentral.com/articles/10.1186/1475-2891-13-61.

Ng, Shu Wen, Meghan M. Slining, and Barry M. Popkin. "Use of Caloric and Noncaloric Sweeteners in US Consumer Packaged Foods, 2005–2009." *Journal of the Academy of Nutrition and Dietetics* 112, no. 11 (November 2012): 1828–34. https://pubmed.ncbi.nlm.nih.gov/23102182.

Nolan, Diana, Jeanne A. Drisko, and Leigh Wagner. *Integrative and Functional Medical Nutrition Therapy Principles and Practices.* Totowa, NJ: Humana Press, 2020.

Pizzorno, Joseph E., and Michael T. Murray. *The Encyclopedia of Natural Medicine.* New York: Atria Books, 2012.

Rakel, David. *Integrative Medicine.* Philadelphia: Elsevier, 2017.

Ruiz-Ojeda, Francisco Javier, Julio Plaza-Díaz, Maria Jose Sáez-Lara, and Angel Gil. "Effects of Sweeteners on the Gut Microbiota: A Review of Experimental Studies and Clinical Trials." *Advances in Nutrition* 10 (January 2019): S31–48. https://pubmed.ncbi.nlm.nih.gov/30721958.

Samsel, Anthony, and Stephanie Seneff. "Glyphosate's Suppression of Cytochrome P450 Enzymes and Amino Acid Biosynthesis by the Gut Microbiome: Pathways to Modern Diseases." *Entropy* 15, no. 4 (April 2013): 1416–63. https://www.mdpi.com/1099-4300/15/4/1416.

Shan, Zhilei, Colin D. Rehm, Gail Rogers, et al. "Trends in Dietary Carbohydrate, Protein, and Fat Intake and Diet Quality among US Adults, 1999–2016." *Journal of the American Medical Association* 322, no. 12 (September 2019): 1178–87. https://jamanetwork.com/journals/jama/fullarticle/2751719.

Trumbo, Paula, Sandra Schlicker, Allison A. Yates, and Mary Poos. "Dietary Reference Intakes for Energy, Carbohydrate, Fiber, Fat, Fatty Acids, Cholesterol, Protein and Amino Acids." *Journal of the American Dietetic Association* 102, no. 11 (November 2002): 1621–30. https://pubmed.ncbi.nlm.nih.gov/12449285.

Wing, Rena R., and Suzanne Phelan. "Long-Term Weight Loss Maintenance." *American Journal of Clinical Nutrition* 82, no. 1 (July 2005): 222S–225S. https://pubmed.ncbi.nlm.nih.gov/16002825.

Zhu, Baoli, Xin Wang, and Lanjuan Li. "Human Gut Microbiome: The Second Genome of Human Body." *Protein & Cell* 1, no. 8 (August 2012): 718–25. https://pubmed.ncbi.nlm.nih.gov/21203913.

RECIPE INDEX

CONVERSIONS

VOLUME

US	US EQUIVALENT	METRIC
1 tablespoon (3 teaspoons)	½ fluid ounce	15 milliliters
¼ cup	2 fluid ounces	60 milliliters
⅓ cup	3 fluid ounces	90 milliliters
½ cup	4 fluid ounces	120 milliliters
⅔ cup	5 fluid ounces	150 milliliters
¾ cup	6 fluid ounces	180 milliliters
1 cup	8 fluid ounces	240 milliliters
2 cups	16 fluid ounces	480 milliliters

US	METRIC
½ ounce	15 grams
1 ounce	30 grams
2 ounces	60 grams
¼ pound	115 grams
⅓ pound	150 grams
½ pound	225 grams
¾ pound	350 grams
1 pound	450 grams

TEMPERATURE

FAHRENHEIT (°F)	CELSIUS (°C)
70°F	20°C
100°F	40°C
120°F	50°C
130°F	55°C
140°F	60°C
150°F	65°C
160°F	70°C
170°F	75°C
180°F	80°C
190°F	90°C
200°F	95°C
220°F	105°C
240°F	115°C
260°F	125°C
280°F	140°C
300°F	150°C
325°F	165°C
350°F	175°C
375°F	190°C
400°F	200°C
425°F	220°C
450°F	230°C

ACKNOWLEDGMENTS

First, I would like to thank my family and friends for jumping back on this book-writing train with me for a second time. We had many déjà vu moments along the way. None of this would have been possible without their enduring love and support. The year 2020 has been one hell of a ride for us all (meaning the entire planet). Having an opportunity to write a second book has been a welcome distraction that provided a silver lining to a dark year.

I'd like to thank the team at Ulysses Press. It's again been an honor and a pleasure to work with you.

ABOUT THE AUTHOR

Dr. Dana M. Elia, DCN, MS, RDN, LDN, FAND, is an integrative and functional nutrition doctor and a licensed, registered dietitian-nutritionist with over twenty-five years of experience. Originally from New Jersey, Dr. Dana relocated to Lancaster, Pennsylvania, in 2001. She is the owner of Fusion Integrative Health and Wellness, LLC, which received the Best of Lancaster award in the nutritionist category in 2019. She is also the author of *The Stem Cell Activation Diet* (Ulysses Press, 2020).

Dr. Dana served as an adjunct faculty member at the Pennsylvania College of Health Sciences and is presently teaching and developing nutrition course curriculums for multiple universities. An active member of her community, Dr. Dana serves on the executive committee of Dietitians in Integrative and Functional Medicine, where she holds the past chair position and previously served as chair, chair-elect, treasurer, and member services chair.

As a recognized leader in integrative and functional nutrition, Dr. Dana has provided content reviews for projects such as the fifth edition of the *Academy of Nutrition and Dietetics Complete Food and Nutrition Guide*. She regularly speaks to both lay and professional audiences and has been featured in, or has authored, numerous articles for *Natural Awakenings Magazine* and *Lancaster Newspaper*.

Dr. Dana's dedication and fervor for the power within food as medicine stems from her own personal journey with autoimmune disease and a rare form of sarcoma. With a passion for ongoing education and a drive to give her patients the best level of care, Dr. Dana completed her doctorate in clinical functional nutrition (DCN) through the Maryland University of Integrative Health, where in 2019 she was awarded the Student Research Poster Award.

In her free time, she loves hiking, camping, kayaking, scuba diving, traveling with her husband James and family, or spoiling her rescued furbabies, Champ, Jasper, and George.